"This book takes a unique multi-disciplinary perspective of the pandemic, reopening strategies highlighting fissures in society and long-held assumptions. The book proposes how universities can lever on management education to help build a resilient and a more inclusive digitally enabled society."

—*Ho Kwon Ping, Founding Executive Chairman of Banyan Tree Holdings and Founding Chairman of the Board of Trustees, Singapore Management University*

I0131839

MANAGING COMPLEXITY AND COVID-19

This book brings together insights and perspectives from leading medical, legal, and business professionals, as well as academics and other members of civil society, on the threats and opportunities to life during the COVID-19 pandemic. It provides a uniquely inter-disciplinary perspective for policymakers, researchers, and medical professionals to assess the different practical strategies, and risk and crisis management processes available to them in addressing the very difficult choices with which they are presented and their implications.

The book presents a framework for the different facets of strategic choices faced by policymakers between life and livelihood, and the challenges of protecting health versus reopening the economy. It also evaluates the intense challenges faced by frontline medical professionals and scientists during an unfolding catastrophe. Finally, the authors explore the societal and human elements of the pandemic and its impact on family dynamics, society, education, and business, including the technology, creative, entertainment, and leisure industries.

This book is deliberately short and captures key insights on the COVID-19 pandemic to form an interdisciplinary overview for professionals, policymakers, and business leaders to consider the long-term implications of the pandemic and lessons for future crises.

Aurobindo Ghosh, PhD, MS (Finance), MStat, Corresponding Editor, Assistant Professor of Finance Education, Director, Citi-SMU Financial Literacy Program, Lee Kong Chian School of Business, Singapore Management University, Singapore. Prof Ghosh teaches and has published peer-reviewed research papers, chapters, and case studies in financial economics and analytics.

Amit Haldar, MD, DM (Neurology), Ex-Fellow of Clinical Neurophysiology, Children's Hospital Boston, USA. Dr Haldar is presently a Consultant Neurologist in India, with special interest in epilepsy and has contributed many book chapters and scientific publications in neurology. His research interests include clinical studies, neurological complications, and the testing of COVID-19.

Kalyan Bhaumik, BA, LLB (Calcutta), Advocate of Supreme Court of India and High Court, Calcutta, Ex-President Rotary Club of Calcutta Old City, India. Advocate Bhaumik practises law in civil and criminal matters, including corporate law, family law, marriage and divorce law, media, entertainment, and sports law, and has authored articles in legal and business economic matters.

MANAGING COMPLEXITY AND COVID-19

LIFE, LIBERTY, OR THE PURSUIT OF HAPPINESS

Edited by
Aurobindo Ghosh, Amit Haldar, and
Kalyan Bhaumik

Routledge
Taylor & Francis Group

LONDON AND NEW YORK

Cover image: Partha Bhattacharjee

First published 2023
by Routledge
4 Park Square, Milton Park, Abingdon, Oxon OX14 4RN

and by Routledge
605 Third Avenue, New York, NY 10158

Routledge is an imprint of the Taylor & Francis Group, an informa business

© 2023 selection and editorial matter, Aurobindo Ghosh, Amit Haldar, and Kalyan Bhaumik; individual chapters, the contributors

The right of Aurobindo Ghosh, Amit Haldar, and Kalyan Bhaumik to be identified as the authors of the editorial material, and of the authors for their individual chapters, has been asserted in accordance with sections 77 and 78 of the Copyright, Designs and Patents Act 1988.

British Library Cataloguing-in-Publication Data
A catalogue record for this book is available from the British Library

Library of Congress Cataloging-in-Publication Data
A catalog record has been requested for this book

ISBN: 978-1-032-11193-3 (hbk)
ISBN: 978-1-032-11516-0 (pbk)
ISBN: 978-1-003-21880-7 (ebk)

DOI: 10.4324/9781003218807

Typeset in Bembo
by codeMantra

Access the Support Material: www.routledge.com/9781032115160

To all the frontline doctors, nurses, essential workers toiling in challenging conditions, to the students who are struggling in the new normal and finally, to the friends and relatives whom we have lost due to COVID-19.

CONTENTS

CONTRIBUTORS

Taimur Baig, PhD, Managing Director, Group Research and Chief Economist, DBS Bank. Previously, Dr Baig served as Principal Economist, Monetary Authority of Singapore (2017), Chief Asia Economist, Deutsche Bank (2007–2017), and Senior Economist, IMF (1999–2007), Singapore. Dr Baig has published widely in specialties including International Finance, Macro-Forecasting and Surveillance, Macro-Financial Linkages, Digital Currency, Climate Change, Productivity, and Innovation.

Hon'ble Justice Debangsu Basak, LLB, Judge, High Court of Calcutta, India. He practised for 21 years principally in the High Court at Calcutta, Company Law Board (Kolkata and New Delhi), Board for Industrial & Financial Reconstruction and Debts Recovery Tribunal specializing mainly in company matters. He was elevated to Additional Judge before being appointed as Permanent Judge.

Alok Bhatt, MD, Pulmonology, Fellow at NYU Grossman School of Medicine, is a specialist in Critical Care medicine and sleep medicine is academically active with research interest in Critical Care medicine and Pulmonary care among others.

Satarupa Bhattacharjee, MSc, IIT Kanpur, B. Sc. obtained her BSc degree, St. Xavier's College, Kolkata, India, both in Statistics, is a PhD candidate in UC Davis under Professor DeaHans Mueller. Her research interests include nonparametrics, Functional Data Analysis, and its overlap with metric geometry, for analyzing functional and non-Euclidean data with applications in brain imaging studies, child neurological development, network analysis.

Ajay Bhattacharya, B.Eng., MBA, Diploma in Directorship, Managing Director at Fortrec Chemicals & Petroleum Pte Ltd, Shareholder, Singapore. Mr Bhattacharya looks after the entire business activities of the group. He has been serving the community in various capacities and received numerous awards and recognitions including the Public Service Medal.

Suborno Bose, PhD, Chairman, IIHM & Indismart Group Worldwide. CEO, International Hospitality Council, is a passionate Hospitality evangelist who founded the world-class IIHM Hospitality Campuses and founded Young Chef Olympiad with over 50 countries taking part.

Subhobroto Chakroborty, Founder and CEO, The Digital Guy is a Digital Marketing Guru who is invited to teach in different business schools in India. Mr Chakroborty also authors online articles on different aspects of digital marketing and impact of the pandemic.

Somnath Chatterjee, MBBS, Co-Founder and CEO, Suraksha Diagnostics, has been managing a multi-modality Diagnostic chain including Radiology & Pathology.

Sanjay Chaudhuri, PhD (Statistics), MStat, BStat (ISI). Prof Chaudhuri is Associate Professor in the Department of Statistics and Applied Probability at the National University of Singapore. Prof Chaudhuri's research interests include Development and Analysis of Statistical Methodologies, in particular based on Empirical Likelihood, Analysis of Complex Survey Data, Order Restricted Inference, Graphical Markov Models, Survival Analysis, etc.

Sushmita Roy Chowdhury, MBBS, MD, Director Pulmonology, Fortis Hospital, Kolkata, is a Pulmonologist passionate about ensuring dignity in suffering.

Sunanda K. Datta-Ray, Journalist and Author, Former Editor of *The Statesman*, and Editorial Consultant, Singapore Press Holding, Singapore. Besides writing for *International Herald Tribune* and *Time*, Mr Datta-Ray was Editor-in-Residence at the East–West Center in Honolulu. He authored books on India and the United States, and won the Vodafone Crossword Book Award LKY's Mission India.

Himanshu Deshwal, MD, Pulmonary and Critical Care Fellow at NYU School of Medicine, is currently pursuing fellowship in Pulmonary Diseases and Critical Care Medicine fellowship at NYU Grossman School of Medicine is academically active with career goals to be an interstitial lung disease and pulmonary hypertension specialist.

Sourav Ganguly, President of the Board of Control for Cricket in India and a former captain of the Indian Cricket team, India. He was a left-handed batsman and captained the Indian national team. He was the President of the Editorial Board with Wisden India and the Cricket Association of Bengal.

Arnab Ghosh, MBBS, MD, Assistant Professor, Department of Virology, PGIMER, Chandigarh, Punjab, India. Dr Ghosh was an Assistant Professor of Microbiology in a Children's Hospital in New Delhi, India. Dr Ghosh has published extensively in medical journals and earned him a Young Scientist member by European Society of Clinical Microbiology and Infectious Diseases.

Kapil Goyal, PhD, is an Associate Professor in the Department of Virology, PGIMER and has numerous publications with respect to COVID-19 research.

Randeep Guleria, MD and DM, has been a Professor and Head, Department of Pulmonary Medicine and Sleep Disorders and Director of All India Institute of Medical Sciences (AIIMS), New Delhi, where he has been working for the last 30 years. Dr. Guleria is the first Indian to get a Doctorate of Medicine (DM) in Pulmonary and Critical Care Medicine. He has done pioneering work in respiratory medicine and COVID-19 response. For his work and contribution to Medicine, in 2015, Dr. Guleria was conferred "Padma Sri," the third highest civilian honor from the Government of India.

Lily Kong, PhD, MA, President and Lee Kong Chian Chair Professor of Social Sciences, Singapore Management University, Singapore. Prof Kong, selected as Forbes top 25 business women in Asia, received several awards including the Fulbright Fellowship Award. She serves on many editorial boards and researches on religion, cultural policy, creative economy, urban heritage, and national identity.

Shuting Liao is a PhD candidate in Biostatistics at the University of California, Davis, under the supervision of Prof. Fushing Hsieh and Prof. Debashis Paul. She is interested in statistical modeling, inference and machine learning.

Vikramjit Mukherjee, MD, Assistant Professor, NYU Grossman School of Medicine, Director, Medical Intensive Care Unit (MICU), Bellevue Hospital Center, NYC, USA, Fellow (NYU Hospitals Center, Pulm & Critical Care, 2015), USA. Vikramjit Mukherjee is the Director of the Medical ICU at Bellevue Hospital, the oldest public hospital in the United States, and the tertiary referral center for New York City's public health system. His research interests lie in emerging diseases.

Rajesh Ranjan Nandy, PhD, Associate Professor of Biostatistics and Epidemiologist, School of Public Health, University of North Texas, USA. Professor Nandy's primary research goal is to develop novel, intuitive, and practical statistical methods to solve real-life problems. The motivation for most of his methodological research comes from real data where conventional statistical approaches are inadequate.

Sovan Patra, PhD, Adjunct Faculty in Singapore Management University. Dr. Patra teaches courses in economics and philosophy. His research reflects a deep and abiding interest in understanding all strains of socio-cultural phenomena.

Debashis Paul obtained his PhD in Statistics from Stanford University in 2005. He completed his BStat and MStat from the Indian Statistical Institute. He is a Professor of Statistics in the University of California in Davis. Prof Paul's research interests include Multivariate Statistics, Random Matrix Theory, Neuroimaging, and Spatial Statistics.

Mini P. Singh, PhD, Professor in Virology, PGIMER, Chandigarh has been involved in outbreak investigations of different viruses and has mentored many labs in North India for COVID-19 testing.

Anurag Srivastava, IAS, Director, MSME and Director Textiles, West Bengal, India. A mechanical engineer from the prestigious Indian Institute of Technology, Kanpur, Mr Anurag Srivastava is an officer at the Indian Administrative Services (IAS) and was in charge of the Directorate of MSME enterprises as well as textiles in West Bengal. He writes commentary in leading media outlets.

Howard Thomas, DSc, PhD, MBA, MSc, Professor Emeritus of Strategic Management and Management Education, Singapore Management University, Singapore. Prof Thomas is a highly cited scholar, whose recognitions include fellowships, and Richard Whipp Lifetime Achievement and Strategic Leadership awards from professional management bodies including the Academy of Management. He has served in senior leadership positions in several universities and global professional management bodies, and is the recipient of several honorary degrees.

FOREWORD: STRATEGY AND MANAGEMENT PERSPECTIVE

From a historical viewpoint, economic crises, epidemics, pandemics, and the spread of infectious diseases have been quite common events. For example, COVID-19 is one of a number of coronavirus-type infections, such as SARS (the Severe Acute Respiratory Syndrome in 2003 in China and Asian countries) and MERS (the Middle East Respiratory Syndrome in 2012 in Saudi Arabia and the Arabian Peninsula), which spread aggressively in those regions. Indeed, some elements of this current global pandemic can even be traced back to the Great Influenza in the early part of the twentieth century which had three waves, the second of which was more devastating than the first (Barry, 2005). Yet, it appears that the strategy and policy-oriented learning about the impacts of the 1918–1919 pandemic, sometimes called "the Spanish Flu" or "The Bombay Fever" (Singh, 2021), might not have been fully absorbed by current global public health authorities. These lessons learned from history might have reduced some of the suffering of people under COVID-19, so history clearly matters! It seems that impacts from the more regional experiences of SARS, MERS, etc. may not have been widely shared despite the fact that South East Asian countries and regions, such as Singapore and Hong Kong, had previously adopted public health measures such as face masks and social distancing to deal with the ongoing coronavirus-type infections and mutations.

The initial stimulus for this book was the co-authors' close examination of the effects of two, "once in a century" global recessions over the last decade. The first, a different type of crisis, was the Global Financial Crisis (GFC) that befell the financial world from 2008 to 2010. While the financial world recovered much faster through coordinated government actions, the consequent disruption of the economy and employment resulted in a much longer recovery period from the ensuing Great Recession (McCorkell and Hinkley, 2019). There was substantial governmental and corporate learning from the GFC, reflected in the changing regulatory structure for financial institutions, increased global cooperation among Central banks, and greater awareness of financial inclusion (Demirgüç-Kunt et al., 2017). However, a missing link was a detailed assessment of individual accountability for the crisis, probably because the main contributory factors for the GFC were identified largely as multi-disciplinary failures of corporate and societal governance. With this background, the authors believe that a multi-disciplinary approach to crisis management situations, incorporating a thorough assessment of individual behaviour, was essential to address the complexity of management problems that policymakers are encountering in today's global pandemic and its much more volatile environmental conditions. These crisis management approaches should enable policymakers to devise future strategies for economic and societal growth.

Why did these authors write this book from this interdisciplinary and behavioural perspective? What was their motivation? One clue is that they were all in high school together in India and remained close friends during their subsequent career journeys in medicine, law, and academia. So, Dr Amit Haldar (Consultant Neurologist), Advocate Kalyan Bhaumik (Practicing Lawyer, The Supreme Court of India), and Assistant Professor of Finance Aurobindo Ghosh at Singapore Management University chose careers in three disparate disciplines. But they had one more thing in common—they all had a global policy "mindset" with India as a specific area of expertise. They fundamentally believed that civil society would be a better place if experts could communicate with one another across professional boundaries and offer broader perspectives and policy options for public policy and crisis management. This was the real impetus that led them to develop and co-edit this volume on Managing Complexity and COVID-19.

It is argued that the Great Influenza (or so-called "Spanish Flu") in 1918 started most probably in Kansas (USA) and might have been a watershed moment for medical education and medical research in the United States (see Barry, 2005). It is perhaps not by accident that the United States is an important contributor to the charge for therapeutics and vaccines for treating COVID-19. In India, where the virulent second wave in 2021 might have been the result of a lax attitude to public health during the pandemic, the situation almost mimicked what happened over a 100 years ago when returning soldiers came back to Mumbai with "Spanish Flu" from their assignment in World War I.

This volume suggests that the current, oft-repeated life vs. livelihood debate might be too simplistic because it leads inevitably to the question: "Whose life is it, anyway?" While such a narrowly framed question and a public discourse is probably more palatable to a news-hungry media, it is apparent that policymakers and expert commentators tend to suffer from an illusion of control while involved in an unexpected, multigenerational crisis event. The progress of science, particularly medical science, to successfully address the current pandemic has been enabled by substantial and risky private sector investment globally in conjunction with publicly funded research institutions. This public–private partnership has discovered therapeutics and vaccines at a pace that has baffled even experts, and clearly the political establishment. The medical profession together with the scientific community has been on the frontline in this current crisis in developing therapeutics, providing medical care, and also defending against sometimes rampant misinformation campaigns conducted in social media often for reasons of political expediency.

The current pandemic has clearly been a disruptive societal force and has stimulated significant changes in many areas including higher education, and particularly in professional management education, with the rapid adoption of technology-enabled online learning. International universities that have managed to pivot teaching approaches towards hybrid and technology-enabled teaching models, as well as being responsive to the needs of the students and other stakeholders, have identified meaningful pathways for improvement. Further, the growth in data-dependent, data analytic policymaking, be it in economic development, public policy, or public health mandates like mask wearing, social distancing, testing, or vaccination-induced herd immunity, has been invaluable in moving to a safer, more secure, and financially included post-pandemic world.

Life as we know it has changed, and might change even more significantly in the future. For example, the practice of law and justice, both in the realms of family and criminal law, with more use of technology-enabled solutions, might make jurisprudence more empathetic and accessible to the masses in India. And in business contexts, all industries dependent on the quick movement of goods and services have been confronted with challenges and supply short-ages in existing global supply chains often resulting in difficulties and production bottlenecks. Policymakers have become more aware also of the problems faced by Small and Medium Enterprises (SMEs), which have been strongly affected by movement restrictions and safe management practices. The collection and dissemination of news stories has also seen a sea change particularly with an onslaught of misinformation (e.g. about vaccine effectiveness) in online false-hoods across social and electronic media platforms, often with polit-ical overtones. Finally, safe distancing and management practices endorsed by medical doctors have significantly reduced perfor-mances of live events including sports and the performing arts. Par-ticularly impacted are young athletes and performers whose career choices in their fields of interest have been adversely impacted by continued restrictions. All these restrictions have hindered the short-run evolution, and futures, of many industries and businesses, but have highlighted the need for the creation of innovative policy alter-natives for achieving sustainable long-term economic growth.

This book is therefore a laudable and perhaps unique attempt to hold up a mirror to society by examining a time capsule of problems faced, decisions made, and actions taken. It aims to capture alterna-tive perspectives on the pandemic and its aftermath from the realms of medicine, business, academia, and civil society to learn about, and reflect on, this multigenerational, wake-up call. This endeavour aims to present a "360 degree" view of facets of the pandemic objectively from various experts, thus helping to restore our faith in hard-earned scientific, medical, legal, and experiential knowledge that may her-ald a more collaborative and cohesive future in this turbulent and complex world.

Prof Howard Thomas,
Former Dean and Emeritus Professor of Strategy
and Management
Lee Kong Chian School of Business
Singapore Management University
12 July 2021

REFERENCES

Barry, J., (2005), *The Great Influenza: The Epic Story of the Deadliest Plague in History*, New York: Viking: Penguin Group.

Demirgüç-Kunt, A., L. Klapper, D. Singer, S. Ansar and J. Hess, (2017), "The Global Findex Database: Measuring Financial Inclusion and the Fintech Revolution," Report, The World Bank Group.

McCorkell, L. and S. Hinkley, (2019), "The Post-Recession Labor Market: An Incomplete Recovery," Report, Institute for Research on Labor and Employment (IRLE), UC Berkeley.

Singh, M., (2021), "Bombay Fever/Spanish FLU: Public Health and Native Press in Colonial Bombay, 1918–19," *South Asia Research*, 41:1, pp. 35–52, doi:10.1177/0262728020966096.

FOREWORD: MEDICAL PERSPECTIVE

"That men do not learn very much from the lessons of history is the most important of all the lessons of history." – Aldous Huxley

It was the year 1918. A devastating influenza pandemic, erroneously named, "The Spanish Flu" struck the world. Modern microbiology was then at its infancy. The causative organ was erroneously suspected to be "Pfeiffer's bacillus" (Eyler, 2010). The real culprit, the influenza virus was too small to be seen by the available microscopes of the time. Many vaccines were tried. All failed. The actual causative organism was neither known nor could it be isolated. People were not aware of its zoonotic origin. At least 50 million people perished in that pandemic all across the globe.

Move forward 100 years. The winter of 2019 saw a similar outbreak starting from the Wuhan city of China. This time modern medical science was more prepared. The causative organism was identified within weeks by advanced techniques of molecular biology and found to be a RNA virus belonging to the Coronavirus family. Vaccines that were safe and effective were developed at breakneck pace. But that was only one side of the story. If we go by the current estimate, almost 5 million people have already died in this pandemic so far (Worldometer, 2021).

Despite the giant strides of modern medicine, we are still searching for an effective treatment for this highly infectious and lethal disease (Lahariya et al., 2020). There are also long-lasting effects of the disease on the body and mind that we are struggling to understand (Taquet et al., 2021). This might have a deep impact on society at large in the days to come.

The present predicament raised certain unpleasant questions. This was not the first pandemic that humans faced. Yet, most of us were not adequately prepared. A woefully low budgetary expenditure in some developing countries on health for decades bears silent testimony to misplaced government priorities. Vaccination programs of various countries have also brought into focus the gross global inequality. Covax, the global vaccine sharing alliance attempting to distribute vaccines worldwide, has altered due to production problems, export ban, and vaccine hoarding (Holder, 2021).

This is where the book *Managing Complexity and COVID19* may have an important role to play. It is a sincere endeavour to look at the present pandemic holistically. A. Ghosh, A. Haldar, and K. Bhaumik, the three editors with different areas of specialization, have managed to rope in experts of various fields ranging from medicine, business, economics, education, law, and sports to share their perspective of this pandemic. In the process, they have attempted to put together the pieces of a jigsaw that can be used to solve similar puzzles of the future.

In the medical section, there are four chapters which look at four different aspects of the disease diagnosis and management. A. Haldar delves into the evolution of the testing process, highlighting the pros and cons of each test. Moreover, he touches upon the unmet needs and how each country has strategized their testing process (Haldar, Chapter 2.1).

R.R. Nandy deals with the mask mandate. Using the example of two counties of the United States, he shows the clear benefit of enforcing a strict mask mandate in reducing the spread of the infection statistically. A simple tool if used properly can have enormous benefits. This should have been enforced earlier. Individual freedom of course gets restricted. But this is a relatively small price to pay for saving precious human lives (Nandy, Chapter 2.2).

Mukherjee et al., in their view from the frontline, paint a poignant picture of the New York City as it faced the first devastating onslaught of the pandemic in the spring of 2020. They have not only highlighted the geographic and demographic factors that led to the spread, but also stressed on the social and economic aftermath that followed. Tales of human triumph amidst the adversities keep our morale up. Shortfall of Personal Protective Equipments (PPEs) round the world draws our attention to keep things ready before hand (Mukherjee et al., Chapter 2.3).

Ghosh et al. dwell on the burning topic of herd immunity. They elaborate on the Great Barrington Declaration to focus protection on the vulnerable population. They also state that while optimum immunization is an important step in containing the disease, this may not be sufficient to end the disease. COVID-appropriate behaviour has to be followed. Otherwise, fresh outbreaks can occur due to waning immunity with passage of time or emergence of a mutant strain (Ghosh et al., Chapter 2.4). Their hypothesis has been borne out by the recent outbreak in Singapore. There the maximum number of daily cases have been reported as late as in October 2021 (when almost 85% of the population is vaccinated along with concurrent safe management measures) (Channel News Asia, 2021). Even the latest case surge in UK has been attributed to waning immunity from vaccination. (Stokel-Walker, 2021)

There are two additional conversations. In one Dr Roy Chowdhury deals with the therapeutic aspects of the management of COVID-19 including the controversy with numerous unproven prophylactic agents. She also touches upon the emergence of an opportunistic secondary fungal infection called Mucormycosis in India. In the second conversation, Dr Chatterjee, a co-owner of one of the leading laboratory chains of India, elaborates how they continued to function 24 by 7 as samples kept increasing day by day. The main challenge was to keep a control over the quality and keep the turn around time (TAT) short.

All in all, the common thread that connects these scientific topics of knowledge about the disease is the multipronged approach to save human life. Globally, the healthcare workers worked day in and day out disregarding their personal safety. Kolkata and New York are just two examples. The book presents an enthralling saga of trials and tribulations that goes beyond scientific or medical data and touches on human relations. It can arouse interest of any serious reader. It also lays down a framework on how to handle future pandemics.

The contributors and the editors need to be congratulated for their combined effort. This book is comprehensive and will remain a testimony for what the world went through in 2020–2021. This will remain a lesson for posterity.

Dr Randeep Guleria
Professor and Director,
ALL India Institute of Medical Sciences
New Delhi
Nov 17, 2021

REFERENCES

Channel News Asia, (2021), "Singapore's Daily COVID-19 Cases Breach 5,000-Mark for the First Time; 10 More Deaths," *CNA Online*, Updated Oct 28, 2021, https://www.channelnewsasia.com/singapore/covid-19-new-cases-deaths-moh-oct-27-2272231, accessed Oct 29, 2021.

Chris, S.-W., (2021), How Bad Is the UK's Covid Situation? *BMJ*, 375:n2597, doi:10.1136/bmj.n2597.

Eyler, J. M., (2010), "The State of Science, Microbiology and Vaccines Circa 1918," *Public Health Reports*, 125:3, pp. 27–36, doi: 10.1177/0033 3549101250S306.

Holder, J., (2021), "Tracking Coronavirus Vaccinations around The World," *The New York Times*, Updated Oct 28, 2021, https://www.nytimes.com/interactive/2021/world/covid-vaccinations-tracker.html, accessed Oct 29, 2021.

Lahariya, C., G. Kang and R. Guleria, (2020), *Till We Win: India's Fight against the COVID-19 Pandemic*, Gurgaon: Penguin Books.

Taquet M, Q. Dercon, S. Luciano, J. R. Geddes, M. Husain and P. J. Harrison, (2021), "Incidence, Cooccurrence, and Evolution of Long-COVID Features: A 6-Month Retrospective Cohort Study of 273,618 Survivors of COVID-19." *PLoS Medicine*, 18:9, p. e1003773, doi:10.1371/journal.pmed.100377.

Worldometer, (2021), "COVID-19 CORONAVIRUS PANDEMIC," Oct 29, 2021, https://www.worldometers.info/coronavirus/, accessed Oct 29, 2021.

PROLOGUE: THE IMPOSSIBLE TRINITY IN A PANDEMIC

Life, Liberty, or the Pursuit of Happiness

INTRODUCTION

On the 4th of July, 1776 the fledgling Congress adopted and ratified the United States Declaration of Independence from the British Empire. This also created a future roadmap for the US Constitution and the Bill of Rights, the birth of an idea for the world's oldest democracy. The inalienable human rights enshrined in the declaration and guaranteed by the founding fathers of this nascent democracy included, among others, "Life, Liberty and the Pursuit of Happiness". Little did they know or envisage nearly 245 years later, in 2020, these three inalienable rights will be in conflict with one another and take the world order to an existential crisis. Governments, policymakers, medical professionals, scientists, academics, and the concerned civil society would be destined to debate this impossible trilemma on the menu of life: "Life, Liberty or the Pursuit of Happiness?"

ASSUMPTIONS: MOST AT RISK FROM THE PANDEMIC

COVID-19, a global pandemic of Biblical proportions with over 4 million deaths (till July 2021), has exposed almost every assumption and every fault-line of the building blocks of our society. In the backdrop of this global malaise, affecting almost every country and continent on the face of the planet, we witness a melange of opposites. Some countries and regions that seem to have successfully negotiated the initial outbreak seem to be falling back into strict lockdowns (e.g., in Asia-Pacific and Africa), while those that struggled initially seem to be coming out of it stronger (e.g., in North America and Europe). Effective vaccines that usually take decades to develop were approved and deployed in 12 months. Despite the miraculous development of immunization, and its scientifically proven effectiveness against severe illness and mortality, vaccine hesitancy, resistance, and nationalism have not waned significantly across the planet and withstood the onslaught of science and logic. The majority of the evolutionary microbiologists have believed that any new infectious agent tending to cause human disease will become less virulent with time, if it has to remain relevant. But some, like microbiologist Andrew Read of Penn State University, said that it is not a universal truth, "It can get nice, and it can get nastier" (Holmes, 2020). The Delta (B1-617-2) variant, possibly the main reason for the surge of cases in India, during the second wave, and fast becoming the dominant strain globally, has demonstrated that higher transmissibility might not mean less virulence. Reopening strategies not cognizant of the nature of the virus can potentially be deleterious to life and livelihood both (Godlee, 2021b, Chapter 1.1).

The origin of the virus is as much shrouded in mystery as the virus itself (Godlee, 2021a). The origin of the novel Coronavirus of the SARS family is attributed to *zoonotic* (from animals to human) transmission, typically from a bat through an intermediary (perhaps, pangolin?) to human. However, since the outbreak recorded in the Huanan Seafood market in Wuhan, China, investigators were baffled as similar virus among bats could not be found in a 1,000 miles radius of the origin. Moreover, the changes that appear in the spike protein of SARS-Cov2 are not present in the Coronavirus affecting bat or pangolin.

One reason for the extremely fast paced development of the vaccines against the virus, particularly the *mRNA* vaccines, was that the entire genome sequence of SARS-CoV-2 was identified and posted online by Chinese researchers on January 10, 2020 (Tufekci, 2021). Science has no religion, no nationality, no borders, and no parochialism. If this is not an example of that, we do not know what is.

The conventional wisdom among climate scientists has often been it was not possible to reduce global greenhouse gas emissions without drastically reducing and transforming economic activity which needs a multi-country agreement like the Paris Climate Accord (COP 21). However, when COVID-19 hit, every country went into a lockdown on their own accord, and this had a significant reduction in green-house gas emissions, both from less vehicular traffic and industries. Despite factory closures, the stock market, which reflects the long-term prospects of the economy, saw one of the strongest runs in recent memory and ended in historic highs. Reining in climate change and economic growth are not mutually exclusive!

Pandemic induced traditional institutions, like the US Supreme Court, to allow oral arguments by phone, a historic first. Despite low internet penetration rates, technological solutions were also pervasive not just in classrooms but also in the courtrooms of India. Like most industries, financial institutions, such as banks, adopted work-from-home arrangements, enabling a flexible environment for mothers of young children to remain in the labour force. This also led to rethinking potentially transformative changes in Universities and Business Schools of the world, making them future ready and more inclusive. Small and medium enterprises (SME) rose to the challenges by pivoting to technology-enabled solutions that led to a boom period for logistics, delivery, and ecommerce spaces, in the midst of general gloom.

Last but surely not the least, research, practice, and deployment of medicine possibly changed for good as well. From the onset of COVID-19, an assumption was made, with scant evidence, that young people are not severely affected by the disease. This is not borne out by the figures in India. Over 40% of the fatalities due to COVID-19 in the All India Institute of Medical Sciences (AIIMS), New Delhi, was of the age group 18–50 years, between April and July 2020 (The Statesman, 2021). Even children were not immune. A multisystem inflammatory syndrome in children (MIS-C) associated with COVID-19 has been reported 4–6 weeks after the occurrence of COVID-19, probably due to a different antibody response or neutrophil extracellular traps (NET) (Jiang et al., 2020).

CONCLUSION: MANAGING COMPLEXITY WITH SIMPLE NARRATIVES

We are humbled by the enormity of information and expertise in areas that are affected by this pandemic. Our objective in this book is to provide a time-capsule of strategy, decisions, and human conditions, with the help of business leaders and professionals, observing policymakers and the evolving paradigm. We delve into the realms of society, economy, medicine, and academia steeped in the complex ecosystem of a global pandemic.

We explore the strategies for making a university future ready, uncovering the asset value of management education, empathetic and sustainable economic policies, and data-driven policy on lockdowns and social distancing, or managing a billion-dollar sports league. We also delve into describing testing protocols and procedures, enforcing of a mask mandate, dispensing emergency medicine in an inequitable society, analysing the truth about achieving herd immunity, processing enormous workload in a medical lab, and discussing issues and benefits of therapies. Finally, our aim is to find solace within families in forced isolation, deep socio-political impact during the pandemic, making SME's to ward over these troubled times, either as a policymaker or as a business leader, educating recruits in the hardest hit hospitality industry, or looking at a boom time for digital marketing.

The biggest challenge of the pandemic is to maintain clear communication and rational thought. Communication from the policymakers to the public, medical professionals to policymakers and finally from the citizens to their government (by their votes if not their voices). NY Governor Andrew Cuomo during his daily briefs in 2020 said something profound. He confided, when he announced the state-wide lockdown, he was morbidly afraid, and two "what if scenarios" kept him up at night. What if the public do not follow the guidance and more scarily, and what if the medical professionals followed the advice and stayed home? Fortunately, neither of these scenarios transpired. Rationality won. New York State, despite being the worst affected in the United States initially, did manage to largely flatten the curve.

We will conclude by reminding the readers of a story about a social scientist who invited a few children in a village to a race to a box of chocolates. It turned out the children held each other's hands and walked slowly to pick up and shared the chocolate bounty.

When asked, a little girl in the race responded, "…how can I be happy when my friends are unhappy?" This concept of *Ubuntu* (from a South African Zulu/Xhosa term) means "…I am because we are," a concept of humanity that resonates with wearing face masks to protect others and maintaining physical distancing, particularly to protect the more vulnerable.

Just imagine, policymakers sometimes have to "mislead" the public, claiming the mask protects you more than others, or incentivise the stronger to get vaccinated to achieve herd immunity to protect the vulnerable. Wouldn't the earlier imaginary story of a little African girl or the real story of the migrant girl in India who bicycled her indisposed father home 1,200 km away be good enough?

Or maybe we should remind ourselves of one of the oldest written quotations in the world, "Vasudhaiva Kuṭumbakam" (Sanskrit phrase in the oldest book known to mankind, the *Vedas*), which simply reminds us "The World is One Family."

REFERENCES

Godlee, F., (2021a), "Covid 19: We Need a Full Open Independent Investigation into Its Origins," *BMJ*, p. 374, doi: 10.1136/bmj.n1721

―――― (2021b), "Caution, Vaccines, Testing: the Only Way Forward," *BMJ*, p. 374. doi: 10.1136/bmj.n1781 (Published 15 July 2021)

Holmes, B., (2020), "How Viruses Evolve," *Knowable Magazine*, Smithsonianmag.com, 17 July, 2020, https://www.smithsonianmag.com/science-nature/how-viruses-evolve-180975343/.

Jiang, L, K. Tang et al., (2020), "COVID-19 and Multisystem Inflammatory Syndrome in Children and Adolescents." *Lancet Infectious Diseases*, 20(11), pp. 276–288, doi: 10.1016/S1473-3099(20)30651-4

The Statesman, (2021), "At 42%, AIIMS Study Finds Highest ICU Mortality among 18–50 Age Group," https://www.thestatesman.com/india/42-aiims-study-finds-highest-icu-mortality-among-18-50-age-group-1502976718.html.

Tufekci, Z., (2021), "Where Did the Coronavirus Come From? What We Already Know Is Troubling," *The New York Times*, June 25, 2021, https://www.nytimes.com/2021/06/25/opinion/coronavirus-lab.html?action=click&module=Opinion&pgtype=Homepage.

ACKNOWLEDGEMENTS

This book would not have been possible without the support and encouragement of several exceptional individuals—colleagues, friends, collaborators, and supporters. We would like to give a shout-out to the incomplete list of inspirations that made this book possible. Prof Howard Thomas has been a constant inspiration for this project even when it was just a fledgling idea. We would like to express our deepest gratitude for all the contributors who took their precious time to work on the chapters despite their extremely busy schedule including SMU President Prof Lily Kong, we are truly humbled. We are also indebted to Dr Randeep Guleria, Director of the All India Institute of Medical Sciences (AIIMS), for authoring the foreword from a medical perspective despite his very busy schedule. We are thankful for conversations with Prof Sanjay Chaudhuri, Dr Taimur Baig at DBS, Mr Gautam Banerjee, Mr Ajay Bhattacharya, and other colleagues at SMU Lee Kong Chian School of Business, Center for Management Practice, Office of Corporate Communications, Executive Education, Library, and Sim Kee Boon Institute for Financial Economics, among others.

We would like to express our deepest gratitude to Ms. Khyati Chauhan for providing exceptional research and editorial assistance. Our gratitude goes to Rebecca Marsh and Manjusha Mishra and team at Taylor and Francis for being so considerate in very challenging times.

The inception of the book transpired over four decades back for all the co-editors attending South Point High School. The friends and classmates have been an enormous source of support. We would particularly like to thank Aparna and Sanjay Das for reaching out to

Sourav Ganguly, to whom we are also indebted to for finding the time to respond to our questions. For various roles the co-editors would like to acknowledge and express thanks to Subhobroto Chakroborty and the Digital Fellow team, Soham Chakraborty, Adam Chua, Anuradha Chatterjee, Chandra Gunawan, Shirley James, Dr Arijit Biswas, Dr Arindam Ghosh, Dr Abhirup Sirkar (Suraksha), Dr Aparajita Chatterjee, Dr Dipanjan Sirkar, Dr Gunjan Gupta, Dr Meena, Dr Abhik Mukherjee and Lynne Thomas, among many others. One special thanks go to renowned artist Mr Partha Bhattacharjee for his creative depiction of Managing Complexity and COVID-19 on the cover.

Last but not the least, we would like to express our heartfelt gratitude to our parents (Samar Kanti Ghosh, Krishna Ghosh, Dr Ajit Halder, Joyanti Halder, Lt Ranjit Bhaumic, and Sabita Bhaumic) for their faith and unconditional blessings, and our spouses (Swastika Ghosh, Lira Haldar, and Anuradha Chatterjee), and our children (Debora Ghosh, Soham Haldar, and Sharanya Haldar) for putting up with our long hours of writing, editing, and meetings for the book often late into the night.

DISCLAIMER

PART I

STRATEGY IN A PANDEMIC

Financial Economics of the
Strategic Choices

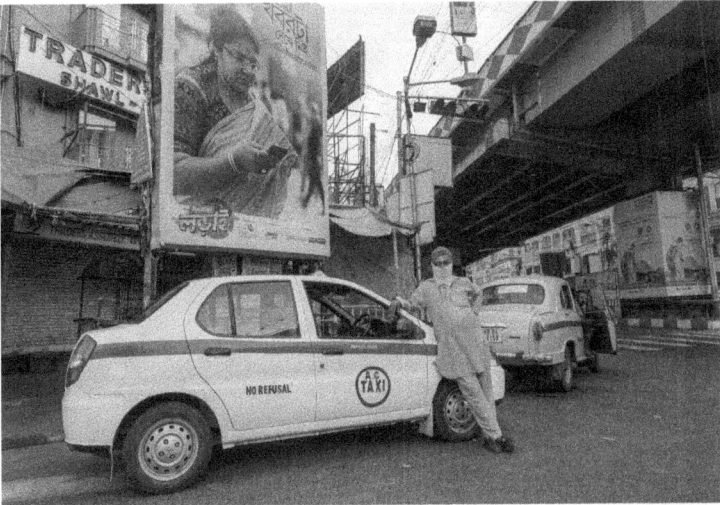

STRATEGIC DEBATE ON FINANCIAL INCLUSION: IS LIFE OR LIVELIHOOD A *FALSE* CHOICE?

Aurobindo Ghosh

...Four historic crises. All at the same time. A perfect storm.

The worst pandemic in over 100 years. The worst economic crisis since the Great Depression.

The most compelling call for racial justice since the 60s. And the undeniable realities and accelerating threats of climate change.

So, the question for us is simple: Are we ready?..

– Democratic Presidential Nominee (and now President) Joe Biden reflected on a US or maybe a global challenge (Pramuk, 2020)

INTRODUCTION

In March 2020, at the onset of the global pandemic Dr Anthony Fauci, Director of the US National Institute of Allergy and Infectious Diseases (NIAID) and later the Chief Medical Advisor for the Biden Administration, when asked about the progression of the virus gave a prophetic response, "...the virus will make the timeline..." (LeBlanc, 2020). Surprisingly, this was one of the very few accurate long-term predictions about COVID-19 made by many experts including Dr Fauci, a 2007 National Medal of Science award-winning scientist and a lifelong public health professional.

DOI: 10.4324/9781003218807-2

In June 2021, more than one and a half years since the virus was first identified in Wuhan, China, many countries were suffering through multiple waves with new more transmissive variants of SARS-CoV-2, causing massive losses of life and livelihood. These "variants of concern" became dominant strains affecting billions, including several children in India who were left orphans by the catastrophic second wave (Ghosh et al., 2021; Kottasova, 2021; Mohan, 2021).

With scant prior data available, policymakers have to make decisions under uncertainty and rely on experts for guidance, often prioritizing the societal benefit and minimizing cost with simulations projecting the impact of the pandemic using epidemiological, economic, and statistical forecasting models (Rowthorn and Maciejowski, 2020, Bhattacharjee et al., 2022). Framing the right question to address this novel threat has engulfed policymakers and concerned citizenry of over 200 countries in all 7 continents on this planet.

When and how can policymakers reopen the economy for the maximal benefit to the society? How can an accurate societal cost–benefit analysis be formulated when the cost is borne by a different group (i.e. the vulnerable immune-compromised older population) and the benefit might be enjoyed by a different group (e.g. the socially isolated, financially excluded, mentally fragile youth)?

There were few predictable or discernable patterns among affected countries or their affected citizens. For example, they range from affluent northern Italy despite having low population density and great medical facilities (Horowitz, 2020) to the care homes in the United States accounting for nearly one-third of the COVID-19 deaths with only 4% of cases (The New York Times, 2021), as well as some of the poorest in shantytown or *favelas* in Brazil having suffered untold devastations (Teixeira, 2021). The virus in this dubious respect has been a "great leveler." This only reflects how helpless policymakers are even with the "ex ante" best-laid plans, when pitted against the vagaries and the wrath of nature. However, technological advancement with the development of vaccines has helped tremendously. During the Great Influenza pandemic (Spanish Flu) more than 100 years earlier the mortality rate (675,000 deaths among 105 million or about one-third of the current US population) was roughly 0.64% or about three to five times the mortality rate in the current pandemic in the United States (Ewing, 2021).

Before the advent of effective vaccines or therapeutics, most Western and developed countries relied heavily on lockdowns alongside social distancing, hand washing, and mask wearing as mitigation measures to contain the outbreak, while applying stimulus spending to supplement lost income (Bhattacharjee et al., 2022).

However, in a developing country like India, the problem is exacerbated by the financial exclusion of the unbanked or underbanked population. On one hand, there are very few social support systems in many developing countries where direct cash transfers to the underprivileged are possible. Therefore, prolonging the lockdown beyond a certain point would render the economically weaker section of society to become truly vulnerable. On the other hand, the premature lifting of the lockdowns to open the economy can often lead to a surge of cases which overwhelm the existing health structure as was evident from the outbreak of the apocalyptic second wave in India.

In this chapter, we make a humble attempt to assess a range of strategic alternatives available to policymakers. However, we will focus only on one narrow slice of this complex jigsaw puzzle. This is the challenge faced by leaders in designing and implementing an effective response to the crisis, despite having access to all the predictions, analyses, and advice provided by scientists, medical professionals, as well as economists. Most countries including those in the Americas, Europe, Australasia, and Asia, including Singapore and India, are examining which strategic choices to make in a balanced and responsive manner to the challenge of safely reopening their economies. In emerging economies, specifically, it is critical to make sure that those more vulnerable, lacking financial and social inclusion, are handled and cared for sensitively and effectively.

STRATEGIC DECISIONS AND COST–BENEFIT ANALYSIS IN A PANDEMIC

The pandemic-ravaged world is obsessed with handling a strategic imperative: A choice between life and livelihood?

We, however, contend that from a societal perspective, the question "What is more important, life or livelihood?" is a *false choice*. Can you imagine a life without a livelihood or livelihood without life? While the first option strikes at the heart of self-worth and financial inclusion for all members of society, the latter is, of course, an unthinkable choice of societal exclusion condemning the vulnerable to stay under the sword of Damocles. However, policymakers encounter this *false dilemma* when questioned by media, businesses, individuals, and civil society. It poses a no-win situation for them, by narrowly framing the life vs. livelihood objective. Maybe a data-driven approach to strategic decision-making can provide a pathway for policymakers to allocate resources sensibly and efficiently. The main aim is to protect the vulnerable with pre-existing conditions or to rejuvenate the economy to reclaim lost jobs.

The projections made available through applying the University of Pennsylvania Penn Wharton Budget Model (PWBM) Simulator indicated (as of June 22, 2020) that if the baseline policy was kept in place (with reduced social distancing), the United States might be able to save 600,000 jobs at the cost of an additional 49,460 lives (Wharton, 2020). Most US states did not reopen, and between June 22nd and August 24th, 2020, the actual counts of death, related to COVID-19, in the United States were approximately 54,228 (Our World In data, 2020), while the number of jobs created (seasonally adjusted employment levels) was approximately 4.4 million (BLS Data viewer, 2021), which when compared to a similar period in 2019 was a much higher number than the PWBM projections (CDC, 2021b). The stronger growth of the job market than that predicted by the model might be attributed to a variety of reasons despite the number of additional deaths predicted being close to the actual number.

DBS-SKBI Singapore Index of Inflation Expectations (SInDEx) Survey of 500 Singapore residents in September 2020 found that around 80% of respondents believed that policymakers should prioritize life over livelihood in the short run, particularly of the vulnerable populations, even at the cost of short-term economic pain before reopening the economy. However, the survey also reported thrice as many respondents preferred reopening at all costs compared to those who wanted to save lives at all costs (SMU, 2020).

Policymakers, who have to weigh in the under-represented but vulnerable population, may consider the maximum probability of loss of life when the economy is reopened, keeping the more costly or Type I error low. They may also try to limit to a benchmark death rate of a vulnerable group from infectious and age-related diseases. Once that is fixed at a low level (say, 0.4% which is the *case fatality ratio* according to US CDC, 2021a), they can focus on minimizing the probability of a less expensive error, like the loss of jobs (the less costly or Type II error), by restarting the economy with appropriate safe management measures. The main data-driven, decision-making tools at the disposal of policymakers are metrics like the basic reproduction rate (or R_0) which measures the number of people infected by each infected person or the test positivity rate in the community (Ghosh et al., 2022).

So, what is the appropriate trade-off between lives and livelihood? In Table 1.1, we help encapsulate a baseline decision-making problem for future resource allocation.

The impact of the infections goes beyond the losses of life. Debilitating organ damage in the form of lung fibrosis, myocardial injury, and brain "fog" has resulted in an evolving syndrome of "Long Haul Covid" (Johns Hopkins Medicine, 2021). Another strategic blunder is the unfettered often exponential propagation of the disease to

Table 1.1 Decision-making under uncertainty at period t. It schematically represents the probabilistic cost–benefit analysis keeping Type I error between 0.4% at case fatality ratio and 20% which according to the September 2020 DBS-SKBI SInDEx survey polled the percentage of citizens who wanted to open the economy at all costs

Policymakers' decision (period t)	*a. Unknown states of nature (period t + 1)*	
	COVID-19 prevalent (COVID)	*COVID-19 dissipated (NO COVID)*
Do Not Reopen Economy (Save Life)	Correct Decision P(Do not Reopen | COVID)	Type II Error (Less Costly Error) P(Do not Reopen | NO COVID) = P(Not reopening economy when threat has subsided)
Reopen Economy (Save Livelihood)	Type I Error (More Costly Error) P(Reopen | COVID) = = P(Reopening economy Prematurely when threat is present) = between 0.4% and 20%	Correct Decision P(Reopen | NO COVID) = Power of the test

achieve "herd immunity" without vaccination that led Sweden to substantially more mortality than its neighbours (Claeson and Hanson, 2020, Bhattacharjee et al., 2022). This might, though inadvertently, also lead to the arrival of more transmissible or virulent variants of the disease and, thus, have dysfunctional impacts on public health (Reicher et al., 2020).

The cost of not reopening is quite detrimental to the long-term sustainability of the society and the economy, particularly impacting the youth, minorities, and female sectors of the population. Delay in reopening the economy may result in many women, with family responsibilities and mostly employed in weakened sectors like retail, tourism, and hospitality, losing their jobs and increasing the gender pay gap ("she-cession") (Holpuch, 2021). The brunt of a stuttering job market might also be felt by younger people whose mental health might already be quite fragile because of an enforced lockdown period (Manji, 2021). Further, the WHO/UNICEF warned of an alarming decline in regular vaccination for other illnesses (WHO, 2020) affecting 23 million children that might precipitate other preventable future outbreaks, while there was a surge in dengue cases in South East Asia during the intermittent lockdowns (Huang, 2020).

The cost of a shutdown (lockdown) of the economy while intended to save lives might not achieve its targets without empathetic treatment of its citizens. For example, the unrest in the United States even before the contentious Presidential elections included the Black Lives Matter (BLM) movement and mounting discontent with several instances of alleged police aggressiveness against minority youths as well as the brutal and needless death of George Floyd while in police custody. There is a growing sense of social injustice and allegations of systematic racism (Tiefenthäler et al., 2020). Further, minority and immigrant communities, particularly Asians, were living in fear as they bore the brunt of increased xenophobia and socio-political vilification (Ruiz et al., 2021).

Following the political polarization that preceded, and reached a crescendo, with the US Presidential elections, unrest did not subside but flared up, ending in the storming of the US Capital on January 6, 2021, for the first time since 1814 (McGreevy, 2021). While developed countries suffered from unrest over issues of historical injustice and racism as well as teenage and adult mental health problems, developing countries suffered from social and economic exclusion triggered by, for example, farmer's unrest in India against new market access laws (Yueng, 2021), and youth unrest in some South East Asian countries (e.g. Thailand, Myanmar). The pandemic might not have caused unrests, but it catalyze them.

The final part of the cost is the deleterious effects of the pandemic on societal, economic, and medical inequality, crowding out the inhabitants in the bottom of the pyramid from resources, causing widespread protectionism and financial exclusion (Piketty, 2019; Thomas and Hedrick-Wong, 2019). Unlike the 1918–1919 Great Influenza that increased inequality, it is estimated that the Black Death plague epidemic in the 14th century, that decimated 50% of the population in Europe, might have significantly affected the lower strata of the society. This led to temporary but macabre reduction in inequality with widespread death among the poor (Alfani, 2021). The international COVAX program, started in 2020, was an attempt for medical equity and solidarity to enable global access to vaccines for the underprivileged communities in the spirit of "one-for-all and all-for-one." However, it has been stuttering, partly due to poorer nations on the largesse of richer countries, who themselves are suffering from rampant vaccine hesitancy (Usher, 2021). Waiting for a vaccination for residents of poorer countries is truly a double-edged sword. On one side, strict social distancing restrictions are bringing in untold hardships to low-middle income households. On the other, in countries with historically low investment in healthcare compared to GDP, like India, those who are getting afflicted with the disease are often pushed into poverty and in financial ruins paying medical bills (Thakur, 2021).

In sum, while many factors impinge upon strategic decisions in pandemic situations, it is vital for policymakers to balance all the direct and indirect costs for both imposing a national or a localized lockdown against the economic growth from reopening their economies (Bhattacharjee et al., 2022).

FACTORS FOR IMPLEMENTING POLICIES: HOW NOT TO LOSE BOTH LIVES AND LIVELIHOOD

What factors would policymakers choose if they prioritize life over livelihood? What factors would those policymakers choose if they prioritize livelihood over life? Are there choices or factors that can lead to loss of both lives and livelihoods? How can policymakers choose options wisely that may save both lives and livelihoods?

Both lives and livelihood could be saved with a ubiquitous world-wide deployment of effective vaccines or therapeutics. In the absence of established therapies for COVID-19, certain combinations of drugs and steroids have been found to have some recuperative benefits (Haldar, 2022). However, widespread availability of vaccines have always been the focus of most pandemic recovery strategies. That is, however, easier said than done. Despite tremendous progress through "Moonshot" discoveries in vaccine development, and lightning speed production absorbing significant strategic financial risk, the deployment of vaccines both within and across boundaries has been far less than ideal. Dr Tedros Adhanom Ghebreyesus, Director-General of the WHO, decrying "trickle down vaccination" pleaded with the international community to share the vaccines to inoculate 10% of the population of each country by September 2021, prioritizing the front-line workers and the most vulnerable before vaccinating the low-risk groups (Clarke, 2021). Countries in South East Asia very effectively dealt with initial phases to keep case count low, but only to resort to heightened alert and restrictions with the rise of more community cases later, and an inadequate rollout of vaccines. As Singapore's National University Hospital Senior Consultant in Infectious Diseases Dr Dale Fisher opined, "…Eventually borders will give way…It's statistically inevitable…" (Pierson et al., 2021).

The main reasons that both lives and livelihood can be lost is possibly fivefold—nature, complacency, negligence, lack of preparedness, and failure to adhere to sound scientific principles. Of the five, the first one is the only one beyond the control of policymakers (a truly external risk) and has been discussed in the introduction. Let's delve into the other four mostly preventable or strategic risks, acknowledging that without having suffered from previous significant outbreaks, expertise in dealing with novel crises is often in short supply in some countries (Kaplan and Mikes, 2012).

However, for both traditional and novel crises, developing capacity is critical for preparedness and subsequent response. Many governments, both local and national, might have been complacent or misguided about their preparedness for the next crisis when the case counts declined. This automatically made them more vulnerable, if and when, subsequent waves of infection arrived. With large developing countries, like India and Brazil, with the second and third highest number of stated infections (and reverse order in deaths, till May 2021), there are some similarities and differences. Historically, investment in healthcare and related infrastructure have been lagging in India with less than 1.3% of GDP coming from government and a total expenditure of 3.6% (out of pocket and public spending), which is significantly low compared to other OECD countries (at 8.8%) and compared to Brazil (9.2%) (Mehra, 2020).

After the first wave subsided, policymakers in India could have been more vigilant before relaxing social distancing, both political and social congregation, and mask wearing mandates, besides upgrading facilities like oxygen generation plants and hospital capacity. When the "tsunami of infections" in the second wave arrived, the country was not ready in time for its second wave effects where oxygen shortage contributed to several avoidable losses of life (Ghosh and Nair, 2020). However, the state of Kerala in India which had the first COVID-19 case in January, 2020, managed to put a system of testing and tracking of patients and supplies in place, along with a network of healthcare workers even after being pummeled by the second wave and currently has one of the country's lowest mortality rates at 0.4% (Bhagat, 2021).

Indian policymakers took the first wave of COVID-19 quite seriously and implemented one of the strictest lockdowns at the initial outbreak in March 2020 (Gettleman and Schultz, 2020). This might have helped reduce the number of deaths significantly and might have also pushed back the second wave compared to the 1918 Influenza outbreak. If it was more complacent about defeating the first wave of the virus in India, it might have been more negligent in Brazil. Administration in Brazil, however, did not take the disease that seriously initially with a lackadaisical attitude towards enforcement of mask wearing and vaccination, which might have led to the world's second largest number of recorded deaths, till May 2021 (Nugent, 2020).

Many countries in the Asia-Pacific and Africa took the learning and experience from previous outbreaks of SARS, MERS, H1N1, and Ebola in the past seriously and instituted standard operating procedures (SOPs) to address the next crisis. These countries and administrative regions including the so-called Asian Tigers, like South Korea, Taiwan,

Singapore, and even some countries in Africa like Uganda were better prepared when COVID-19 arrived on their shores (although many had to revert to localized lockdowns). However, countries in Europe, the Americas, and South Asia were often caught under-prepared.

Finally, despite an incredible feat of discovering several different safe and efficacious vaccines besides some therapies, there has been a concerted effort to undermine these scientific advances. Some are probably due to naiveté (e.g. uninformed or misinformed anti-vaxxers), but some others are intentional with more selfish interests (e.g. covert business or political interests). Some politicians and administrators might have intentionally or inadvertently planted seeds of vaccine hesitancy and resistance alongside doubts about certain public health measures like social distancing and mask wearing. Some promoted unproven, often dangerous, therapies and strategies in association with inaccurate statements like "...Children almost never transmit the disease...." (Flaherty, 2020).

SOCIETY AND SOCIAL MEDIA: WEAPONIZING DISINFORMATION OR FALSEHOOD

The element of the pandemic that cannot be understated is the role of social media, not only for its informational value but also unfortunately in weaponizing dissemination of falsehood propagating unproven treatments and few anti-vaccine campaigners fomenting vaccine hesitancy through falsehoods and by overemphasizing rare side effects (CCDH, 2021).

For example, social media was an important influence in the second wave in India where scarcity of oxygen and critical care hospital beds led to significant number of avoidable deaths. Social media empowered the concerned citizenry to provide support and information on availability and access of oxygen supply in a woefully unprepared country of 1.35 billion, and these actions overwhelmed the under-funded government infrastructure (Lyons, 2021).

However, the dark side of social media (as well as some traditional media) came out in the proliferation of fake news and falsehood about therapeutics and vaccines, both in terms of access and efficacy (The Straits Times, 2020). While some of the falsehood might have been unintentional, nefarious and opportunistic actors furthered their business and political interests by sowing seeds of discontent and divisiveness, and exploited the vulnerability of the uninformed and fearful population through social media, despite regulators like the FDA's efforts to stop them (Rosenbaum, 2020).

CONCLUSION: ONLY TOGETHER WE (MIGHT) STAND

Having discussed these strategic challenges, we cannot be proactive in a dynamic world without recognizing that the virus is evolving continuously with new variants posing new challenges around the world including varying efficacy of vaccines (Zimmer, 2021). Even with developed countries like the United States and the United Kingdom, which can potentially afford to continue with a longer-term lockdown, the level of pandemic fatigue can potentially prove detrimental to the youth, particularly from the economically and socially vulnerable communities, which may, in turn, lead to street protests about lack of opportunity.

In a novel crisis such as the COVID-19 pandemic, scenario analyses and scenario planning (e.g. Simulation, War Gaming) are required in order to envisage every possibility that was not experienced or even thought of before. What was the likelihood, prior to the crisis, that one of the world's foremost and popular flagship airlines, Singapore Airlines, running nearly to capacity, would have to ground over 96% of their fleet, in a short span of time in March 2020 (Thomson Reuters, 2020)? In a novel crisis, preparedness risk assessment includes the use of horizon scanning to detect emerging threats and engaging experts using multidisciplinary assessment approaches besides healthcare capacity building (Baubion, 2013).

However, we also observe random acts of kindness both from individuals donating much needed oxygen (Mukherjee, 2021; Lee and Morton, 2021) and G7 countries pledging to donate billion dosage of vaccines. These activities result from a greater appreciation of inequality in wealth, both among nations and people, and the consequent need for access for minorities and the disadvantages to vaccine solutions. Despite the proliferation of falsehoods, vaccine nationalism, inequitable access, and pandemic restriction fatigue, we hope to herald a genuine collaborative effort by the countries to engage in devising humane and meaningful solutions to eradicate, conquer, or control the potentially endemic COVID-19 virus.

Indeed, managing complexity and enabling financial inclusion in a pandemic-ravaged world is a challenging task in the *best of times* and possibly futile *in the worst of times*. It is clear that we don't stand a chance unless we stand together to solve crises in this seemingly Dystopian world straight out of a Dickensian novel.

NOTE

This contributed chapter was accepted for publication in this refereed edited volume on June 18, 2021.

REFERENCES

Alfani, G., (2021), "Epidemics, Inequality and Poverty in Preindustrial and Early Industrial Times," *Journal of Economic Literature*, 59:1, pp. 3–44.

Baubion, C., (2013), "OECD Risk Management: Strategic Crisis Management," OECD Report.

Bhagat, S. V., (2021), "As India Stumbles, One State Charts Its Own Covid Course," *The New York Times*, 23 May 2021, https://www.nytimes.com/2021/05/23/world/asia/coronavirus-kerala.html.

Bhattacharjee, S., S. Liao, D. Paul, and S. Chaudhuri, (2022), "Taming the Pandemic by doing the Mundane," In *Managing Complexity and Covid-19: Life, Liberty, or the Pursuit of Happiness*, Edited by A. Ghosh, A. Haldar and K. Bhaumik, Routledge, pp. 62–82.

BLS Data viewer, (2021), "Labor Force Statistics from the Current Population Survey," https://beta.bls.gov/dataViewer/view/timeseries/LNS12000000.

Center for Countering Digital Hate (CCDH), (2021), "The Disinformation Dozen: Why Platforms Must Act on Twelve Leading Online Anti-vaxxers," Mar 2021, https://www.counterhate.com/disinformationdozen, 17 Jul, 2021.

CDC, (2021a), "COVID-19 Pandemic Planning Scenarios," 19 March 2021, https://www.cdc.gov/coronavirus/2019-ncov/hcp/planning-scenarios.html.

CDC, (2021b), "Daily Trends in Number of COVID-19 Cases in the United States Reported to CDC," https://covid.cdc.gov/covid-data-tracker/#trends_dailytrendscases.

Claeson, M. and S. Hanson, (2020), "Covid-19 and the Swedish Enigma," *The Lancet*, 397: pp. 259–261.

Clarke, J., (2021), "As It Happened: Unequal Access to Covid Jabs Scandalous – WHO Chief," *BBC* News, 24 May 2021, https://www.bbc.com/news/live/uk-57225462.

Ewing, E. T., (2021), "Measuring Mortality in the Pandemics of 1918–19 and 2020–21," *Health Affairs*, 1 April 2021, https://www.healthaffairs.org/do/10.1377/hblog20210329.51293/full/.

Flaherty, C., (2020), "Not Shrugging Off Criticism," https://www.insidehighered.com/news/2020/09/23/scott-atlas-white-house-adviser-coronavirus-threatens-sue-colleagues-back-stanford.

Gettleman, J. and K. Schultz, (2020), "Modi Orders 3-Week Total Lockdown for All 1.3 Billion Indians," *The New York Times*, 24 March 2020, https://www.nytimes.com/2020/03/24/world/asia/india-coronavirus-lockdown.html.

Ghosh A. and R. Nair, (2020), "Modi Govt Invited Bids for 150 Oxygen Plants in October. Today, Just 33 Are Up," *The Print*, 24 April 2020, https://theprint.in/health/modi-govt-invited-bids-for-150-oxygen-plants-in-october-today-just-33-are-up/644643/.

Ghosh, A., K. Goyal, and M. Singh, (2022), "COVID-19 Herd Immunity and Role of Vaccines," In *Managing Complexity and Covid-19: Life, Liberty, or the Pursuit of Happiness*, Edited by A. Ghosh, A. Haldar and K. Bhaumik, Routledge, pp. 130–144.

Ghosh, A., W-K. Lim, A. Haldar and K. Bhaumik, (2021), "The Covid-19 Crisis in Thailand: Charting a Safe and Sustainable Path to Recovery," Case No: SMU-20-0041, *Harvard Business Publishing and Singapore Management University*, Center for Management Practice.

Haldar, A., (2022), "Navigating an Unchartered Sea: Finding the Right Test and Testing Pathway," In *Managing Complexity and Covid-19: Life, Liberty, or the Pursuit of Happiness*, Edited by A. Ghosh, A. Haldar and K. Bhaumik, Routledge, pp. 89–111.

Holpuch, A., (2022), "Hiring is Rebounding in the US – But the 'Shecession' Persists," *The Guardian*, 24 April 2021, https://www.theguardian.com/us-news/2021/apr/24/us-hiring-jobs-women-shecession.

Horowitz, J., (2020), "Italy's Health Care System Groans under Coronavirus — A Warning to the World," *The New York Times*, 17 March 2020, https://www.nytimes.com/2020/03/12/world/europe/12italy-coronavirus-health-care.html.

Huang, E., (2020), "Outbreak of Dengue Fever in Southeast Asia Is 'exploding' Amid the Coronavirus Fight," https://www.cnbc.com/2020/07/10/outbreak-of-dengue-fever-in-southeast-asia-is-exploding-amid-the-coronavirus-fight.html.

John Hopkins Medicine, (2021), "COVID 'Long Haulers': Long-Term Effects of COVID-19," *John Hopkins Medicine*, 1 April 2021, https://www.hopkinsmedicine.org/health/conditions-and-diseases/coronavirus/covid-long-haulers-long-term-effects-of-covid19.

Kaplan, R. S. and A. Mikes, (2012), "Managing Risks: A New Framework," Harvard Business Review, June 2012.

Kottasova, I., (2021), "What We Know about the Covid-19 Delta Variant First Found in India," https://edition.cnn.com/2021/06/10/health/delta-variant-india-explained-coronavirus-intl-cmd/index.html.

LeBlanc, P., (2020), "Fauci: 'You Don't Make the Timeline, the Virus Makes the Timeline' on Relaxing Public Health Measures," *CNN*, 26 March 2020, https://edition.cnn.com/2020/03/25/politics/anthony-fauci-coronavirus-timeline-cnntv/index.html.

Lee, J., and B. Morton, (2021), "G7: World Leaders Promise One Billion Covid Vaccine Doses for Poorer Nations," https://www.bbc.com/news/uk-57461640.

Lyons, K., (2021), "Social Media Platforms Become Triage Centers as India Struggles with a COVID-19 Surge," *The Verge*, 25 April 2021, https://www.theverge.com/2021/4/25/22402273/twitter-whatsapp-facebook-triage-center-india-oxygen-hospital-coronavirus.

Manji, H., (2021), "The Growing Mental Health Crisis in the Wake of COVID-19," *The Forum Network*, 21 May 2021, https://www.oecd-forum.org/posts/the-growing-mental-health-crisis-in-the-wake-of-covid-19.

McGreevy, N., (2021), "The History of Violent Attacks on the U.S. Capitol," *Smithsonian Magazine*, 8 January 2021, https://www.smithsonianmag.com/smart-news/history-violent-attacks-capitol-180976704/.

Mehra, P., (2020), "India's Economy Needs Big Dose of Health Spending," *Live Mint*, 8 April 2020, https://www.livemint.com/news/india/india-s-economy-needs-big-dose-of-health-spending-11586365603651.html.

Mohan, R., (2021), "As Parents Succumb to Covid-19 in India, Children Are in Distress," *The Straits Times*, 9 May 2021, https://www.straitstimes.com/asia/south-asia/as-parents-succumb-to-covid-19-in-india-children-are-in-distress.

Mukherjee, T., (2021), "India's Second COVID-19 Wave Sparks Selfless Acts, But the Battle Is Far from Over," https://www.channelnewsasia.com/news/cnainsider/india-second-covid-19-wave-sparks-selfless-acts-battle-hospitals-15013398.

Nugent, C., (2020), "Brazil Is Starting to Lose the Fight against Coronavirus— And Its President Is Looking the Other Way," *Time*, 21 May 2020, https://time.com/5840208/brazil-coronavirus/.

Our World in Data, (2020), "Daily New Confirmed COVID-19 Deaths per Million People," https://ourworldindata.org/explorers/coronavirus-data-explorer?zoom-ToSelection=true&time=2020-03-01..latest&pickerSort=desc&pickerMetric=new_deaths_per_million&Metric=Confirmed+deaths&Interval=7-day+rolling+average&Relative+to+Population=true&Align+outbreaks=false&country=IND~USA~GBR~CAN~DEU~FRA.

Pierson, A., R. Jennings and H. Lowry, (2021), "These Parts of Asia Beat Coronavirus Early. Why They're Suddenly in Lockdown," *Los Angeles Times*, 18 May 2021, https://www.latimes.com/world-nation/story/2021-05-18/covid-asia-new-lockdowns.

Piketty, T., (2019), *Capital and Ideology* (Translated by Arthur Goldhammer). Cambridge, MA: Harvard University Press.

Pramuk, J., (2020), "Read Joe Biden's Full 2020 Democratic National Convention speech," https://www.cnbc.com/2020/08/21/joe-biden-dnc-speech-transcript.html.

Reicher, S., S. Michie and C. Pagel, (2020), "Covid-19: What Should We Do about B.1.617.2? A Classic Case of Decision Making under Uncertainty," *The BMJ Opinion*, 17 May 2021, https://blogs.bmj.com/bmj/2021/05/17/covid-19-what-should-we-do-about-b-1-617-2-a-classic-case-of-decision-making-under-uncertainty/.

Rosenbaum, L., (2020), "InfoWars Founder Alex Jones Must Stop Selling Fake Coronavirus Silver Cures, FDA Says," *Forbes*, 9 April 2020, https://www.forbes.com/sites/leahrosenbaum/2020/04/09/infowars-founder-alex-jones-must-stop-selling-fake-coronavirus-silver-cures-fda-says/?sh=1ae73626541a.

Rowthorn, R., and J. Maciejowski, 2020, "A Cost–Benefit Analysis of the COVID-19 Disease," *Oxford Review of Economic Policy*, 36:S1, pp. S38–S55.

Ruiz, N. G., Edwards, K. and Lopez, M. H., (2021), "One-Third of Asian Americans Fear Threats, Physical Attacks and Most Say Violence against Them Is Rising," *Pew Research Centre*, 21 April 2021, https://www.

pewresearch.org/fact-tank/2021/04/21/one-third-of-asian-americans-fear-threats-physical-attacks-and-most-say-violence-against-them-is-rising/.

SMU, (2020), "Inflation Expectations Decline with a Rise in Global Uncertainty," 19 October 2020. https://news.smu.edu.sg/news/2020/10/19/inflation-expectations-decline-rise-global-economic-uncertainty.

Teixeira, F., (2021), "Brazil's Favelas Struggle to Count Their Dead as Coronavirus Rages," *Thomson Reuters*, 2 April 2021, https://www.reuters.com/article/us-health-coronavirus-favelas-trfn-idUSKBN2BZ132.

Thakur, A. (2021), "Medical Bills Are Ruining Indians: Ask Amit Paswan's Widow," *The Times of India*, 16 June 2021, https://timesofindia.indiatimes.com/india/covid-killed-amit-paswan-and-condemned-his-family-to-lifetime-of-poverty/articleshow/83429280.cms.

Thomson Reuters, (2020), "Singapore Airlines to Ground Most of Its Fleet as Travel Curbs Bite," *Thomson Reuters*, 23 March 2020, https://www.reuters.com/article/health-coronavirus-singapore-air/singapore-airlines-to-ground-most-of-its-fleet-as-travel-curbs-bite-idUSL4N2BG08I.

The New York Times, (2021), "Nearly One-Third of U.S. Coronavirus Deaths Are Linked to Nursing Homes," *The New York Times*, 28 April 2021, https://www.nytimes.com/interactive/2020/us/coronavirus-nursing-homes.html.

The Straits Times, (2020), "ScienceTalk: Covid-19 Vaccine Facts, Fallacies and Hoaxes," The Straits Times, 7 December 2020, https://www.straitstimes.com/singapore/sciencetalk-covid-19-vaccine-facts-fallacies-and-hoaxes.

Thomas, H. and Y. Hedrick-Wong, (2019), *Inclusive Growth: The Global Challenges of Social Inequality and Financial Inclusion*. Bingley: Emerald Publishing.

Tiefenthäler A., C. Triebert, D. Jordan, E. Hill, H. Willis and R. Stein, (2020), "How George Floyd Was Killed in Police Custody," *The New York Times*, 31 May 2020, https://www.nytimes.com/2020/05/31/us/george-floyd-investigation.html.

Usher, A. D., (2021), "A Beautiful Idea: How COVAX Has Fallen Short," *The Lancet*, 397:10292, pp. 2322–2325.

Wharton, (2020), "Coronavirus Policy Response Simulator: Health and Economic Effects of State Reopenings," 1 May 2020, https://budgetmodel.wharton.upenn.edu/issues/2020/5/1/coronavirus-reopening-simulator.

WHO, (2020), "WHO and UNICEF Warn of a Decline in Vaccinations during COVID-19," https://www.who.int/news/item/15-07-2020-who-and-unicef-warn-of-a-decline-in-vaccinations-during-covid-19.

Yueng, J., (2021), "Farmers across India Have Been Protesting for Months. Here's Why," *CNN*, 26 March 2021, https://edition.cnn.com/2021/02/10/asia/india-farmers-protest-explainer-intl-hnk-scli/index.html.

Zimmer, C., "The World Is Worried about the Delta Virus Variant. Studies Show Vaccines Are Effective against It," *The New York Times*, 6 July 2021, https://www.nytimes.com/2021/07/06/science/Israel-Pfizer-covid-vaccine.html.

UNIVERSITIES IN AND BEYOND A PANDEMIC

Lily Kong and Sovan Patra[1]

INTRODUCTION

Insofar as universities are spaces that depend and thrive on intellectual exchange and collaboration, it is not surprising that COVID-induced restrictions on in-person interactions have had a transformational impact on the way in which they deliver education, and consequently, on students' learning experience. Similarly, research in many disciplines has been negatively impacted due to limited access to facilities (laboratories) while stresses following the rapid shift in the mode of teaching, coupled with increased care responsibilities, have impacted productivity for many faculties and researchers. Student, faculty, and staff well-being have been challenged by the psychological and emotional stresses generated by isolation, the simultaneous obligation to discharge multiple responsibilities, and anxieties about health. At the same time, the unprecedented pandemic-wrought travel restrictions have placed additional financial burdens on universities, and for some, in crisis proportions. Those universities that are agile and can pivot well to address the plethora of challenges stand to last the long haul. For others, decline—swift or slow—will be difficult to reverse for a long time to come.

Entire books could be written about the impacts of the pandemic on universities. The constraints of space in a short chapter prompt us to focus on just two dimensions: the delivery of education and the

DOI: 10.4324/9781003218807-3

financial challenges that universities face. The impacts of COVID-19 on education and finances vary from university to university, system to system, and country to country. In what follows, we highlight some of the more egregious examples, as well as reflect on our own lived experience teaching at, managing, and leading the Singapore Management University (SMU) amidst a pandemic.

TEACHING AND LEARNING IN A TIME OF COVID

Since the WHO decision to declare the COVID-19 outbreak a pandemic in January 2020, public health authorities around the world have, with varying degrees of promptness, seriousness, and success, imposed a variety of restrictions on social interaction, and internal and international mobility. Campus closures at short notice, where they were in term, implied that universities had to migrate, impromptu to remote learning platforms. The challenges involved in such mass migration have been helpfully categorized as technological, pedagogical, and social (Ferri et al., 2020).

The technological challenge lay in ensuring equitable access to academic content for the student population and ensuring secure and seamless content delivery. Ensuring equitable access is challenging for two reasons. In developing countries, such as Pakistan (see Adnan and Anwar, 2020), where there is differential access across the student population to fast and reliable internet services, online teaching can exacerbate, rather than attenuate, socio-economic inequalities. A further source of unequal access to learning is the difference in the home environments that students learn in. Although digital spaces are platforms for interaction between the student and the content, the quality of that interaction is mediated by the physical spaces in which the interaction occurs. Zhang et al. (2020) discuss the problems experienced with disparate home-based learning environments in China's pivot towards remote learning in the early stages of the pandemic. The bottom line is that in the absence of solutions to the problems above, remote learning compromises the potential for university education to drive social mobility.

Concerns of equity aside, the technological challenges in delivering content securely and seamlessly have also been substantial. Remote learning enables access to university servers and databases from relatively less secure home-based networks and devices. Given this additional level of vulnerability and the trend towards increasing sophistication in the modus operandi of cybercrime, preventing data breaches and the sort of malware and ransomware attacks that RMIT in Australia was exposed to earlier in the year, will be key to any successful and sustainable remote learning strategy (ABC News, 2020). Further, given the suddenness of the shift to remote learning, universities have faced an infrastructure (both physical and human) deficit in ensuring seamless programme delivery. Most universities around the world have had some capacity to deliver content online for some time now (although that capacity differs greatly across universities in the economic north and south and even across universities in the same economic region). However, even if this infrastructure would have sufficed for attempts (often token) at incorporating some form of digital instruction in the normal curriculum, Pace et al. (2020) accurately identify that the current circumstances are more appropriately labelled 'crisis-learning,' rather than 'normal digital learning.' In such settings, ensuring that existing or newly acquired infrastructure can cope with the scale of the stress placed on it, and over a sustained period, has been a daunting task.

The pedagogical challenges were similarly multi-pronged: firstly, among faculty, a deficit in digital skills and an enthusiasm to acquire the same quickly needed to be addressed. In addition, the gap in praxis, between making academic content accessible online and ensuring that learning objectives are effectively met through remote instruction, needed to be closed. Rapanta et al. (2020) have argued, in this context, that content designed for delivery in a classroom rarely translates well when delivered remotely. The same is true for activities designed to encourage class participation and group collaboration. One of the authors of this chapter discovered this first-hand, while snooping around 'breakout rooms' in Zoom after students had been assigned an activity to discuss and address as a team. Activities that would elicit active and heated debate in classrooms produced nothing but a lull in breakout rooms. The alienness of content and activities designed for the classroom in a virtual environment was also mirrored in assessment design and implementation. Further, motivational issues (for both students and faculty) stemming from the lack of interactivity in a technology-mediated learning environment needed to be mitigated. These issues are generally attributable to the (missing) general immanence of the classroom space, the (missing) herding effect it produces, and the non-immediacy of the instructor–student interaction (in this last context, Adnan and Anwar (2020) identify lagged feedback from instructor to student as a key impediment to motivation).

The social challenge was in managing the cognitive stresses that prolonged social isolation engendered. This is evident especially in university communities, where meaning of and about the world is created and contested through sustained interpersonal communication, prolonged deprivation of the same can, and is documented to, produce mental distress (see Son et al., 2020; Fruehwirth et al., 2021). Further, Giavimrimis and Nicolaou (2020) have aired anxieties about the dissipation of social capital that campus-based interaction produces among students. The effect of this on social cohesion, student participation in social enterprise, and, more generally, personal well-being is anticipated to be deleterious. In this light, the practical challenge in maintaining university-based social networks has been to find the best proxy for the ideal of campus-based interaction in these non-ideal circumstances.

COVID AND THE FINANCIAL CHALLENGES OF RUNNING A UNIVERSITY

While the curbs on social interaction have challenged universities globally to find ways to sustain the humdrum of university operations, the effects of controlling international travel have been significantly more adverse for some universities, with financial ramifications expected to last beyond the pandemic. For many of these highly 'internationalized' universities, located primarily in anglophone countries, the short- and medium-term stress on finances caused by travel restrictions has been exacerbated by escalating geopolitical uncertainties. But it is worth noting that the pandemic and the geopolitics have only exposed, rather than caused, the underlying, systemic weaknesses in the universities' financial models.

To understand the genesis of the current woes facing many universities, one needs to consider both exogenous factors and an evolution in the way that modern research universities compete. For a start, it is important to recognize that, over the last two decades, there has been a steady diminution in support of the view that higher education is a public good. In public policy, for example, in the

United Kingdom and Australia, this has translated into a reluctance to increase the use of tax revenues to fund teaching and research at universities (Berman, 2012), and indeed, to reverse such use as much as possible. To compensate for the shortfall in budgetary allocation, rules have been relaxed on tuition fee caps for local students and on caps on foreign student enrolment. Increasingly, and in tandem with accelerating globalization, universities have turned to foreign students (who, in many instances, pay significantly higher tuition fees) to manage the twin pressures of a shrinking public purse and a mandate to maintain university education as aspirational and consequently affordable for local students.

The internationalization of the higher education landscape has been driven by other factors and articulated in other ways as well. The increase in the fixed and variable costs of research, in addition to putting further premium on foreign students, has internationalized the competition for research capital; the increase in the number of academics has also internationalized the academic labour market (Musselin, 2018). Further, universities no longer compete solely based on the signalling potential of their degrees but also on the quality of the experience they offer their student bodies. The marketing of education as part-signal, part-investment, and in equal part, consumption (see Ghosh and Thomas, 2022) has in turn increased the pressures for horizontal differentiation. Internationalized campus demographics and the promise of international exchange programmes and internships have become staples in the pursuit of differentiation. Finally, the institutionalization of the competition between universities in the form of league tables and rankings has added further impetus to the push for internationalization in its myriad forms.

Against this backdrop, the protracted restrictions on international mobility have threatened the internationalization project directly, by reducing foreign (both, resident and exchange) student numbers, as well as indirectly. The indirect effect stems from reputation erosion: sustained border closures have resulted in foreign students across the globe struggling with dormitory closures and job losses and being denied the safety valve of a return home. Evidence from Australia to the United States suggests that a large proportion of this class of students has been heavily reliant on financial support (in many cases, for food) from social welfare groups and charitable individuals (Alpert and Nguyen-Feng, 2020; Firang, 2020). With state aid largely restricted to citizens, universities with large foreign student populations are under increasing pressure to intervene on humanitarian grounds, as well as to combat the growing perceptions of disenfranchisement and second-class treatment. The absence of intervention and reputational damage are likely to hinder recovery in foreign student enrolment numbers which, during the pandemic, have fallen off the cliff in many places. In the United States, for instance, foreign student enrolment for the Fall 2020 term recorded a 43% year-on-year decline (Struck, 2020). In Australia, continued border closures are projected to cause a 50% decline in foreign student numbers (Menchin, 2020). While the United Kingdom bucks the trend by posting a rise, there is uncertainty about whether the numbers indicate 'trade creation' rather than 'diversion' (The Conversation, 2020).

The financial impact of closed borders and closed campuses on higher education has been unprecedented. For instance, Nietzel (2020) reports the impact on American colleges and universities at an estimated USD 120 billion. University bottom lines have particularly suffered from the precipitous drying up of revenue streams; dramatic declines in foreign student enrolment have caused equally drastic drops in tuition-related revenue. Universities in Australia (2020), for example, have reported a drop of AUD 1.8 billion in operating revenue in 2020, with a further AUD 2 billion decline projected for 2021. In addition, auxiliary revenues from dormitory rentals, rentals of sports facilities, and from sundry on-campus commerce have also disappeared, as has the revenue from short-term contractual research (Pruvot et al., 2020; Whitford, 2021). On the other hand, university expenditures have also increased substantially. For example, the University of California's Office of Federal Governmental Relations (2020) reported a COVID-driven increase of USD 341 million in direct expenditures (till August 2020). This largely unbudgeted increase has been driven by a plethora of factors, including the need for investment in technology to support remote instruction, the need to implement social distancing and sanitary protocols, the need to provide medical, psychological, and financial support to staff and students, the need to make provisions for tuition and accommodation-related refunds, and the need to honour contractual obligations to compensate for cancelled student trips and programmes. In several instances, higher costs have been driven by idiosyncratic interventions to support and retain existing foreign students and enrol new ones. These incur repatriation costs, quarantining costs, and the costs of chartering planes to bring new students to campus (Bang, 2020; Nott, 2020).

Financially distressed universities and associations across university systems around the world have urgently requested help from the public exchequer. In many such instances, aid of some form has been forthcoming. This aid has either taken the form of direct transfers (as in the case of the United States [Murakami, 2021]), liquidity support by bringing forward tuition payments and access to low interest loans (as in the case of the United Kingdom [Pruvot et al., 2020]) and Australia (Universities Australia, 2020), participation in publicly funded job retention schemes, and commitments to maintain or increase research budgets. The United Kingdom also has a formal restructuring plan for universities at risk of COVID-induced insolvency (Department for Education, 2020).

Nevertheless, the public support packages have generally been inadequate in plugging the short-term hole in university finances. As such, universities have had to resort to streamlining their expenditures, and were cutting or deferring non-essential infrastructure investment has not been sufficient, cost optimization initiatives have entailed cutting personnel costs. Interventions aimed at reducing expenditures on personnel have varied along a continuum of severity; at their most lenient, they have only necessitated hiring and salary freeze (as has been the case with the 'endowed' private universities in the United States [for example, see Molina, 2021]), and at their most severe they have also involved job losses. Australian universities, for instance, have shed at least 17,300 jobs in 2020 (Universities Australia, 2021) and universities in the United Kingdom have cut at least 3000 jobs (McKie, 2020). State universities in the United States and smaller private universities have also borne their share of job cuts (Sainato, 2020). In some instances where universities have avoided large scaling back in personnel numbers, they have had to implement salary reductions (for example, the University of Maryland (2020) has required its employees to take up to a 10% pay cut for the duration of 2021). It is also noteworthy that, where university employment has declined, the data suggest that the most vulnerable in the academic hierarchy have borne the brunt. Adjunct faculty and junior administrators are significantly more at risk of losing their jobs than tenured faculty (Douglas-Gabriel and

Fowers, 2020). This is easily explained by noting that, in general, state-sponsored income support policies allow tenured, but not adjunct, faculty to be furloughed. It also highlights how, even in the higher education sector, the pandemic and interventions to address its impact have exacerbated socio-economic inequalities.

COVID AND SMU: A BRIEF CASE STUDY

We turn now to the impact of COVID-19 on SMU, and through our respective lenses of president and adjunct faculty, recount the challenges and responses. The first COVID-19 case was confirmed in Singapore on 23 January 2020. Universities in the country were forced to respond rapidly in multi-faceted ways. At SMU, as at many other universities, the pandemic thrust colleagues in facilities management, safety and security, and IT into the frontline, with cleaning, maintenance, IT provision, and security becoming critical functions, foregrounding their generally taken-for-granted roles. On campus, cleaning regimes were enhanced, safety and security arrangements stepped up, and, as the campus emptied out, rentals waived for businesses on campus that had to stop their trade. Depending on the vagaries of the situation, split-team work arrangements and safe-working measures have alternated with work-from-home arrangements. A suite of measures was introduced to support faculty and staff, such as providing online health and well-being programmes, offering new online learning and development opportunities, and extending tenure clocks and contract terms for faculty. A COVID-19 microsite providing resources and information for the community was set up to keep faculty and staff fully updated on circumstances and the university's response.

Classes and examinations moved online in a hybrid manner (with some of the class online and others in person) or, when circumstances required, completely online. Student recruitment, orientation, freshmen welcome programmes, graduation ceremonies, and other university events and activities pivoted online at short notice. Even activities that ordinarily require students to carry them out beyond the campus pivoted online: these include virtual internships, virtual real-world 'consultancy' projects (termed SMU-X projects), virtual exchange programmes, and virtual community service activities. In short, the core educational intent has been kept intact and experiential learning has been delivered albeit with a different kind of experience, one that is, perhaps, no less important and useful. For a full semester from January 2021, classes were entirely conducted in person as circumstances improved, but look set to move online again at the point of writing, as apparently more contagious strains of the coronavirus have made their way into Singapore. In the midst of continuous uncertainty, faculty expertise has played, and will continue to play, a key role in undertaking topical research and informing policy on a range of issues including, the impact of isolation on elderly persons, the role of e-retail, the impact and mitigation of logistics and supply chain disruptions, and the safe and humane management of migrant worker dormitories.

The university's efforts to maintain normalcy and contribute to society in testing times has been acknowledged by its own, as well as the larger community. A pulse survey undertaken at the height of the crisis scored SMU 8 out of 10 for rising to address the crisis. Nearly a year later, in another pulse survey, 92% agreed (to varying degrees) that they felt confident that the university was responding well to the challenges posed by the pandemic. To quote one colleague, 'SMU's response to Covid has made me proud to be part of SMU and I can see that students really appreciate the various accommodations that have been made.' In the same year, SMU won national awards and recognition: as among Singapore's best employers and for its creativity in delivering a virtual graduation ceremony. The university also posted an operating surplus despite the challenges.

Even though the world, Singapore, and SMU are not yet out of the woods, lessons learnt from last year will help keep the ship steady for the months (and years) ahead. First, since the SARS (Severe Acute Respiratory Syndrome) outbreak in 2003, SMU has provided training for faculty to deliver classes online in a programme termed Emergency Preparedness for Teaching and Learning (EPTL). When COVID-19 struck, faculty knew what to do, or else, could very quickly refresh their competencies. Even if/when COVID-19 eventually passes, it will not be the last pandemic. The lesson learnt is what the Boy Scouts always knew: 'Be prepared.'

Second, it became apparent through the first semester of teaching during COVID-19 that classes are best held either fully online or fully offline; a hybrid class, with some students online and some face-to-face, is not satisfactory for either group of students, and is much more challenging for faculty. In fact, at SMU, there were many members of faculty who taught entirely online and delivered so effectively that their teaching scores improved. The important thing was to keep true to SMU's pedagogical philosophy, anchored in the conception of the student as an individual and a social being, which translates into using technology to enhance personalized learning and interactive learning, respectively. The latter is especially important; in avoiding the use of asynchronous video lectures and emphasizing, instead, synchronous interaction, discussion, and participation, even when delivering online, many SMU faculty have been effective in their pivot. Since this can be more challenging to facilitate than in in-person discussion, SMU deployed more teaching assistants to support faculty. The remaining challenge is in delivering experiential learning effectively. While there have been some colleagues who have successfully delivered a learning experience that students have appreciated even more than before, the majority of those delivering their courses using SMU-X pedagogy, for instance, have received slightly less favourable feedback than under normal circumstances. We think that the solution lies not in finding increasingly fancier technologies to use, but in using technology creatively to enable experiential learning in unconducive circumstances.

A third lesson from the current pandemic and crisis is the need to 'communicate, communicate, and communicate.' Rumours, misinformation, and fear have a proclivity to fill the gaps created by lack of information. Empathetic listening and demonstration of care and understanding by leaders at every level is very important to keep the morale and team together. If communication is critically important at the level of an organization, it is indispensable at the level of society. In this aspect, the role of the university as a thought leader, and as a bulwark against the proliferation of stubborn ignorance, is invaluable. That role is generally challenged in unprecedented times, such as ours, where experts do not have enough evidence to come to a consensus about what the fact is. The challenge for the university, then, is twofold. It needs to build, among its student population, a resilience to misinformation by making them critical thinkers; in addition, it needs to engender, in its pool of experts, the commitment to a clear, accurate, and accessible articulation of their research agenda and findings.

Fourth, agility in terms of budgetary management is crucial to securing the long-term financial health of a university. The ability and willingness to make appropriate adjustments to expenditures is critical. At SMU, there was a temporary freeze on hiring but a commitment was made not to lay off staff and faculty except for contracts which would have ended regardless. The ability to capitalize on opportunities is equally important—as Singaporeans chose to stay in Singapore for their education instead of going overseas, SMU was fully responsive to the increased demand, and adjusted to ensure that there would be faculty to address teaching needs. At the same time, the growth in demand for continuing education programmes from adult learners looking for short courses to upskill and reskill was anticipated and delivered via the SMU Academy (SMUA). SMUA pivoted very quickly, rolling out new online courses in digitalization, which, in addition to augmenting productivity of individuals and society, increased university revenues (see also Ghosh and Thomas, in this volume). The moral of the story is that universities exist in a symbiotic relationship with society; the greater the social gains they produce, the better off they are, individually.

Fifth, a close (critical but not confrontational) partnership with government agencies enhances the value of universities in uncertain times. The larger national environment, based on this model of collaboration between the government and the higher education sector, enabled universities, including SMU, to operate effectively. Financially, the Job Support Scheme, which contributed towards the salaries of Singaporeans, helped cover some costs that were incurred in dealing with the pandemic. The Ministry of Education and Immigration and Checkpoints Authority worked with universities to ensure that student visas could still be issued, that a system was in place for foreign students to be quarantined upon arrival, and for COVID-19 tests to be administered efficiently. The experience in many parts of the world suggests that none of this integrated approach can be taken for granted.

THE OUTLOOK

How universities teach is unlikely to change in the long term, despite the COVID-induced shift towards remote learning. That said, the once-bitten universities are likely to increase their investment in acquiring a capacity to deliver remote learning at short notice. A by-product of this investment may be that face-to-face classes will harness technology more effectively. In other words, remote, technology-mediated interaction is likely to complement, rather than be a substitute for the physical classroom space.

Further, despite the scale of the current shock to universities' bottom lines, the pandemic is unlikely to have a substantial medium- to long-term financial impact on universities/university systems for several reasons. Firstly, recessions provide an impetus to university enrolment by lowering the opportunity costs of university education (Ghosh and Thoma (2022) also identify the demand for education as counter-cyclical). The growth in enrolment in the United Kingdom, referred to above, supports this hypothesis. Secondly, most university systems have had access to some form of temporary public support, however limited, to mitigate the fiscal effects of the pandemic. Thirdly, data suggest that students prefer being taught in-person rather than virtually, and want to enjoy campus life, with its opportunities for sport, social activity, and residential experience. They are thus keen to return to campuses. This suggests that auxiliary revenues will also recover in the medium term.

So, from a long-term perspective, COVID-19 and concomitant state interventions have merely highlighted the systemic weaknesses in university structures and governance practices, which a changing geopolitical environment will further stress. The unprecedented proliferation of universities and programmes in the first two decades of the 21st century, driven by increasing numbers of foreign students, now—in the light of China–US tensions, and a more general waning in enthusiasm for globalization—appears not only unsustainable but also in need of correction. In other words, there appears to be too many universities, for too few local students, especially in countries with an ageing demographic. For non-elite universities, facing substantial cost pressures, the resulting inability to exploit scale economies can be fatal. Further, in several countries, the downward pressure on enrolment is likely to be exacerbated by scepticism—fuelled as much by the ideological commitments of the populist right, as by pragmatic concerns about the rate of return on the public investment in universities—about the value of a university education. Critiques of the value of university education pose an especially existential threat to departments and programmes in the humanities and the liberal arts, especially in the wake of the pandemic, since the pandemic has highlighted the social value of university-based research in mathematics (epidemiological modelling), sciences (vaccine development), and technology (vaccine and ventilator manufacture and track and trace application development). Indeed, university-related public funding during the pandemic has prioritized either STEM research or vocational programmes (like teaching) that satisfy a national labour need. The humanities in particular, and universities in general, thus need to underline their intangible, non-fungible social value; that lies in teaching students to develop as citizens who are resilient to misinformation and dogma and, thus, are bulwarks against social fragility and monolithism.

Universities, and departments and programmes in universities, are stratified by reputation, by their perceived social value, and by their financial strength (measured, partly, by their access to donations and loans). The elite universities, and the departments/programmes that are perceived to be strategic state assets, by virtue of their signalling potential or state protection, are likely to be relatively insulated from geopolitical and social pressures. The less fortunate face the prospect either of closure or of consolidation unless they successfully remap their relevance to the world they are embedded in.

NOTE

This contributed chapter was accepted for publication in this refereed edited volume on May 28, 2021.

1   All correspondence with respect to this chapter can be directed to Sovan Patra at email: sovanpatra@smu.edu.sg.

REFERENCES

ABC News, (2020), *Melbourne's RMIT University Suspends Classes after Suffering IT Outage*, https://www.abc.net.au/news/2021-02-19/melbournes-rmit-university-suffers-suspected-cyber-attack/13173704, 19 February 2020.

Adnan, Muhammad and Anwar, Kainat, (2020), Online Learning Amid the COVID-19 Pandemic: Students' Perspectives, *Journal of Pedagogical Sociology and Psychology*, 2(1), pp. 45–51.

Alpert, Judith and Nguyen-Feng, Viann N., (2020), COVID in New York City, the Epicenter: A New York University Perspective and COVID in

Duluth, the Bold North: A University of Minnesota Perspective, *Psychological Trauma: Theory, Research, Practice, and Policy*, 12(5), pp. 524–528.

Bang, Xiao, (2020), International Students to Arrive in Australia for First time in Nine Months under Pilot Program, *ABC News*, https://www.abc.net.au/news/2020-11-29/first-charter-flight-international-student-darwin-pilot-program/12928626, 29 November 2020.

Berman, Elizabeth Popp, (2012), *Creating the Market University: How Academic Science Became an Economic Engine*, Princeton: Princeton University Press.

Douglas-Gabriel, Danielle and Fowers, Alyssa, (2020), The Lowest-Paid Workers in Higher Education Are Suffering the Highest Job Losses, *The Washington Post*, https://www.washingtonpost.com/education/2020/11/17/higher-ed-job-loss/, 17 November 2020.

Department for Education, (2020), *Establishment of a Higher Education Restructuring Regime in Response to COVID-19*, https://assets.publishing.service.gov.uk/government/uploads/system/uploads/attachment_data/file/9026f08/HERR_announcement_July_2020.pdf, 16 July 2020.

Ferri, Fernando, Grifoni, Patrizia and Guzzo, Tiziana, (2020), Online Learning and Emergency Remote Teaching: Opportunities and Challenges in Emergency Situations. *Societies*, 10(4), p. 86.

Firang, David, (2020), The Impact of COVID-19 Pandemic on International Students in Canada, International Social Work.

Fruehwirth, Jane Cooley, Biswas, Siddhartha, and Perreira, Krista M., (2021), The Covid-19 Pandemic and Mental Health of First-Year College Students: Examining the Effect of Covid-19 Stressors Using Longitudinal Data, *PLOS ONE*, 16(3), p. e0247999.

Giavrimis, P. and Nikolaou, Souzanna M., (2020), The Greek University Student's Social Capital during the COVID-19 Pandemic, *European Journal of Education Studies*, 7(8), pp. 1–16.

Ghosh, A. and H. Thomas, (2022), "Is Management education a Valuable Long-Lived Financial asset?" In *Managing Complexity and Covid-19: Life, Liberty Or The Pursuit of Happiness*, Edited by A. Ghosh, A. Haldar and K. Bhaumik, Routledge.

McKie, Anna, (2020), UK Universities Axe Thousands of Jobs during Pandemic, *The World University Rankings*, https://www.timeshigher education.com/news/uk-universities-axe-thousands-jobs-during-pandemic, 8 December 2020.

Menchin, Jennifer, (2020), Australia: Covid-19 Restrictions Could Result in 50% Int'l Student Drop, *The Pie News*, https://thepienews.com/news/australia-covid-19-could-result-in-50-international-student-drop-reports/, 17 November 2020.

Molina, Samantha, (2021), University Salary and Hiring Freeze to Be Lifted for the Next Academic Year, *The Guardian*, https://www.browndailyherald.com/2021/02/02/university-salary-hiring-freeze-lifted-next-fiscal-year/, 2 February 2021.

Murakami, Kery, (2021), Billions in Aid Head to Colleges, *Inside Higher* Ed, https://www.insidehighered.com/news/2021/01/15/education-department-releases-billions-aid-colleges, 15 January 2021.

Musselin, Christine, (2018), New Forms of Competition in Higher Education, *Socio-Economic Review*, 16(3), pp. 657–683.

Nietzel, Michael T., (2020), Pandemic's Impact on Higher Education Grows Larger; Now Estimated to Exceed $120 Billion, *Forbes*, https://www.forbes.com/sites/michaeltnietzel/2020/09/29/pandemics-impact-on-higher-education-grows-larger-now-estimated-to-exceed-120-billion/?sh=6d-6f588522bd, 29 September 2020.

Nott, Will, (2020), Universities Consider Charter Flights for International Students, *The PIE News*, https://thepienews.com/news/unis-consider-charter-flights-for-international-students/, 26 June 2020.

Pace, Christi, Pettit, Stacie K., and Barket, Kim S., (2020), Best Practices in Middle Level Quaranteaching: Strategies, Tips and Resources Amidst COVID-19, *Becoming: Journal of the Georgia Association for Middle Level Education*, 31(1), p. 2.

Pruvot, Enora Bennetot, Estermann, Thomas, Kupriyanova, Veronika, and Stoyanova, Hristiyana, (2020), *Public Funding Observatory 2020/2021 Part 1: Financial and Economic Impact of the Covid-19 Crisis on Universities in Europe*, European University Association, https://www.eua.eu/downloads/publications/pfo%20part%201_ppt%20-%20im.pdf.

Rapanta, C., Botturi, L., Goodyear, P., Guardia, L. and Koole, M., (2020), Online University Teaching during and after the Covid-19 Crisis: Refocusing Teacher Presence and Learning Activity, *Postdigital Science and Education*, 2, pp. 923–945.

Sainato, Michael, (2020), Outrage as Coronavirus Prompts US Universities and Colleges to Shed Staff, *The Guardian*, https://www.theguardian.com/

us-news/2020/aug/12/us-universities-colleges-job-losses-coronavirus, 12 August 2020.

Son, Changwon, Hedge, Sudeep, Smith, Alec, Wang, Xiaomei and Sasangohar, Farzan, (2020), Effects of COVID-19 on College Students' Mental Health in the United States: Interview Survey Study, *Journal of Medical Internet Research*, 22(9), p. e21279. doi: 10.2196/21279.

Struck, K, (2020), New International Student Enrollment Falls 43% in the US, *Voice of America*, https://www.voanews.com/student-union/new-international-student-enrollment-falls-43-us, 16 November 2020.

The Conversation, (2020), Why International Students Are Choosing the UK – Despite Coronavirus, https://theconversation.com/why-international-students-are-choosing-the-uk-despite-coronavirus-147064, 7 October 2020.

The University of California's Office of Federal Governmental Relations, (2020), University of California COVID-19 Request Highlights and Update on Expenditures and Lost Revenues, https://ucop.edu/federal-governmental-relations/_files/Advocacy/covid-19/20200930-covid19-updated-expenditures-and-losses.pdf, September 2020.

Universities Australia, (2021), 17,000 Uni Jobs Lost to COVID-19, https://www.universitiesaustralia.edu.au/media-item/17000-uni-jobs-lost-to-covid-19/, 3 February 2021.

University of Maryland, (2020), Financial Impacts during COVID-19, https://umd.edu/virusinfo/emails/091020, 10 September 2020.

Whitford, Emma, (2021), Pandemic's Fall Financial Toll Adds Up, Inside Higher Ed, https://www.insidehighered.com/news/2021/01/12/colleges-spent-millions-covid-19-expenses-fall-even-sources-income-shrank-data-show, 12 January 2021.

Zhang, Wunong, Wang, Yuxin, Yang, Lili, and Wang, Chuanyi, (2020), Suspending Classes without Stopping Learning: China's Education Emergency Management Policy in the COVID-19 Outbreak, *Journal of Risk and Financial Management*, 13(3), p. 55.

THE GLOBAL PANDEMIC AND MANAGEMENT EDUCATION

Is Management Education a Valuable Long-Lived Financial Asset?

Aurobindo Ghosh and Howard Thomas

INTRODUCTION

Even with signs of economic rebound following vaccination drives in many developed countries led by the United States and United Kingdom, the so-called Group of Seven Central Banks around the world have continued to keep their interest rates low (Bloomberg News, 2021) together with accommodative monetary policy and the largest ever stimulus spending the world has ever seen (Ranasinghe and Rao, 2020). One obvious concern that plagued the policymakers, prompting unprecedented monetary and fiscal policy deployment, was the possibility of the collapse of the global economy. Hence, support for businesses was offered so as to protect them from bankruptcy or job retrenchment by using, for example, job support schemes like the UK Furlough (Coronavirus Job Retention Scheme, 2020) and the US Paycheck Protection Program (2020). Further, the 2020 CARES Act provided emergency relief for education, while the American Rescue Plan of 2021 allocated $170 billion for new programme development (CARES Act, 2020). According to a recent McKinsey Report, the stimulus spending as a response to the global pandemic dwarfs the amount spent in the aftermath of the 2007–2008 global financial crisis (GFC) (Cassim et al., 2020).

DOI: 10.4324/9781003218807-4

The main downside risk, which turned out to be unfounded in the wake of widespread fiscal stimulus spending for the GFC, was again, the potential return of inflation risk (Wolf, 2021).

The deluge of global stimulus spending may have simply percolated into asset prices and caused a notable bubble in different asset markets including real estate and cryptocurrencies, besides traditional stocks and bonds (El-Erian, 2021). This "irrational" financial exuberance may of course result in the collapse or "burst of a bubble" of these potentially high-yielding assets.

However, some individual retail investors have searched for assets that might be immune to such short-term "froth" in the market, particularly those that might also be countercyclical or where the demand for the asset would increase when the economy is in a downturn. Such assets may not be tradeable, unlike a stock or a bond, but their value may be long lived. One such asset might be investment in education at a personal or societal level, in order to address the shortage of skills needed to rebuild ailing economies. An example in the education domain could be upscaling human capital in management education, which is an area that often exhibits a higher demand during market downturns and economic disruptions (see, for example, Kong and Patra, 2022). In addition, management education is generally a personalized but a non-tradeable and non-transferrable asset.

IS MANAGEMENT EDUCATION AN INVESTMENT GOOD?

Is there potential value in developing human capital assets in volatile economic environments? Is education an investment good? Can we argue that personal and educational development is a "sensible" investment? Is this a good time for getting management education?

These questions are relevant but nuanced and demand a multi-pronged response. We examine five different observations from financial economics about the supply and demand for education. These issues hold the key to addressing an economic and strategic view of education, particularly in management education (Gordon and Howell, 1959; Schoemaker, 2008; Cornuel et al., 2021).

First, a liberal undergraduate education is considered a universal "right of passage" and deemed to be for personal intellectual development and enrichment (Harney and Thomas, 2020). Hence, as a commodity the "consumption" element is probably more prevalent than the "investment" element. While general undergraduate education can be deemed to be a consumption good, we will separately discuss a special category of highly in demand degrees from elite universities that are sought more for "conspicuous consumption". For example, Professor Scott Galloway of New York University has noted that "Academics and administrators at the top universities have decided over the last 30 years that we're no longer public servants; we're luxury goods" (Walsh, 2020).

However, the impact of the global pandemic on these new graduates might subsequently be felt in a much thinner employment market for younger first-time job seekers, particularly those with very little management experience or training, who might need to signal more clearly their distinctive capabilities (see, for example, Kong and Patra, 2021, in this volume). Demand in the market has shifted towards hiring graduates having a mix of analytical and managerial/administrative skills, since the nature of many of the traditional starting jobs is being disrupted through digital transformation and automation in manufacturing and restructuring of the financial services industry (Frey and Osbourne, 2017).

Second, by contrast, professional management education is often deemed to be an "investment good" rather than a pure "consumption good". Similar to real estate, management education is potentially a "fungible" asset; it is interchangeable as a "consumption" or an "investment" good. While demand for commoditized undergraduate education is likely to be more price inelastic, typically demand for professionally oriented management education might be more price sensitive (price elastic) than undergraduate education with some notable exceptions, i.e. the elite programmes which have a strong brand image or reputation such as Harvard, Stanford, or MIT.

Third, particularly for the so-called elite programmes, graduate as well as undergraduate education might be the purported commodities of "conspicuous consumption" or *Veblen* Goods (Veblen, 1899) where the demand goes up even when the prices go up, *ceteris paribus*, in violation of the standard law of demand which postulates a downward sloping demand curve (The Economist, 2009). Characteristics constituting a Veblen good might be an outcome of two possibly interacting phenomena. First, the "conspicuous consumption" or luxury good part that often involves an "illusion of scarcity" with production controlled like Hermes' Birkin bags or Rolex Daytona Cosmograph watches (Walsh, 2020). Second, an intrinsic value part, an assurance of increasing returns due to brand recognition or prestige that follows graduation from elite programmes. Such elite graduation is generally well rewarded by employers offering a significantly higher stream of future salaries even with less than equivalently higher performance levels (Taras et al., 2020). In a world where prospective investors are seeking higher returns, and in the business school ranking-focused, hyper-competitive "winner takes all" ecosystem described as the "tyranny of rankings" environment this perceived investment value gained through higher post-pandemic employment prospects and salaries may contribute to a higher demand for quality management education (McGee and Thomas, 1986; Pfeffer and Fong, 2004; Policano, 2005; Ghoshal, 2005; Khurana, 2007; Augier and March, 2011; Cattani et al., 2017; Peters and Thomas, 2018; Starkey and Thomas, 2019; Alvarado, Ghosh and Thomas, 2019; AACSB Magazine, 2021; Cornuel et al., 2021).

The fourth element of this discussion revolves around the societal value creation of the graduate management degree based on an ecosystem involving the business student, the management school offering the degree, and the providers or suppliers (most often faculty) who help deliver the management programme. The value created for a management degree is the difference between the prospective students' "willingness to pay" (WTP) the tuition fees (or their reservation price from the demand side) and opportunity cost of the suppliers or the providers for the management school (Brandenburger and Stuart, 1996). Figure 3.1 describes the value chart, where the management student's value created is determined by their WTP, and the tuition and fees charged by the management school. In addition, the value created for the management student comprises the value for "conspicuous consumption" (or the luxury good element) and the intrinsic value dictated by the future stream of income.

However, a return on investment (ROI) argument with the associated measurement of any individual management student's created value is a much more challenging prospect as it involves both subjective or endogenous choice and uncertainty. Brandenberger and Stuart (1996) also contend that in comparison to a firm's behavior and measurement, "...assessing the willingness-to-pay of consumers

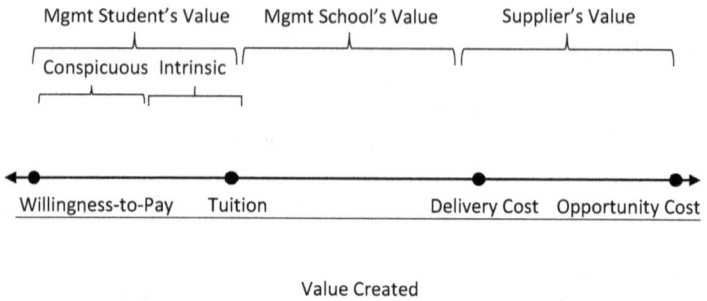

Figure 3.1 The value chart in education process

of household products is often harder". Consumer behaviour suggests that "…perceived value plays a relatively greater role when setting the maximum purchase price whereas reference market prices have greater impact when deciding on the minimum selling price…" (Simonson and Drolet, 2003).

Finally, from the supply side, management (business) schools are in a prime position to grab this opportunity to offer a wider suite of programmes, particularly technology-enabled ones, and at more competitive price points in order to meet the potential burgeoning demand for more competitive fee levels and value. This might lead to a more inclusive management education that can appeal to both managers who are unwilling to relinquish their current jobs (thus reducing the opportunity cost) and prospective managers whose financial accessibility to a management degree may be a difficult issue. From the perspective of the business schools that are just below the elite schools in terms of rankings, this might herald a similar disruption seen by the financial world in the wake of the global financial crisis (GFC) and help them maximize their revenue at lower programme price points through achieving higher student value and enrollment levels. This creative process of matching the demand and supply patterns is likely to enhance the perceived personal investment value of management education.

Rephrasing Billy Joel's immortal song, with respect to the future value of Management Education, COVID-19 "…did not start the fire …," but it surely can help to accelerate a mindset change in which management education is not just an investment good but a new asset class.

TRANSFORMATION OF EDUCATION UNDER COVID-19

According to the World Economic Forum, "…COVID-19 has struck our education system like a lightning bolt and shaken it to its core. Just as the First Industrial Revolution forged today's system of education, we can expect a different kind of educational model to emerge from COVID-19…" (Kandri, 2020).

In the wake of the crisis, all educational institutions starting from primary schools, secondary schools to 2–4-year colleges, universities, and business schools have been forced to adopt distance and remote learning models using enterprise video communication software like WebEX and Zoom. Most dinner tables during the day were converted into teachers' lecterns or students' desks. While this caused incredible disruption and blurred the boundary between home and school or home and work, the empty offices and erstwhile classrooms and executive education centres mandated significant change not only for the education system but also for the mindset of many educational administrators and faculty members.

Hence, we examine the impact of COVID-19 on management education and suggest that it might turn out to be longer lived and even more transformational than changes advocated, but not implemented, by management educators in the first two decades of the 21st century.

As the global economy is teetering unsteadily and inequitably towards normalization, at least in many developed countries, with widespread vaccination and pandemic mitigation measures like social distancing mainly in developing countries, hybrid models—often described as "blended learning"—are rapidly replacing in-person instructional methods in the field of management education. The hybrid model of partly online and partly in-person pedagogical format has inevitably been adopted in undergraduate programmes where there is still a preference for "face-to-face" instruction and to a limited extent in some professional MBA and executive education programmes. The hybrid format has not been fully embraced from either the demand or the supply perspective, yet there are exceptions such as the Instituto De Empressa, Madrid, Spain (or IE)/SMU Blended Learning MBA programme, and IE's successful blended learning programme designs. In addition, there have been new fully online programmes such as in the Questrom School of Business in Boston University (in partnership with ED-X) and the iMBA in the Gies School of Business in the University of Illinois (in partnership with Coursera) that have added considerable creativity in online design, following a string of successes in online or part-time MBA programmes over the last 20 years. Such success stories include programmes in schools such as Warwick (WBS) and Imperial in the United Kingdom, and Indiana (Kelley) and North Carolina (Kenan-Flagler) in the United States (see, for example, the online MBA rankings published annually by the *Financial Times*).

It is important to understand that there have been three major catalysts for adoption of these online or hybrid programmes. First, the tight and competitive job market has meant early career management professionals often between 32 and 37 years age (forming the majority of the registrants or students attending the online MBA programme in the Questrom School of Business in Boston University; see, for example, Poets and Quants, 2021) found it challenging to find time outside of work and family commitments to undertake a fulltime degree (MBA CSEA, 2020). Second, the opportunity cost for these management professionals who wanted to upgrade their knowledge and qualifications was too high when adding the lost opportunity of the existing job besides the substantive fees (of full-time programmes) that often might add on to their already burgeoning student debt. The flexibility that online and hybrid programmes offered was deemed to be quite phenomenal. These programmes could be made fully customizable. For example, experts from different global institutions could potentially deliver the modules, and degrees could be made much more flexible and stackable leading, for instance, to micro-master's degrees earned through completion of each "bite-sized basket" of appropriate modules (for example, a degree in digital business made up of a range of modules in IT and data analytics). This could also enable lifelong learning to flourish and be much more affordable (for example, Executive Education in Gordon Institute of Business Studies (GIBS), University of Pretoria, South Africa or the SMU Academy at SMU).

The obvious question now is, despite all these catalysts with both pull and push factors, why did the hybrid form of education wait for a global pandemic to be considered as a serious educational option? Inertia, institutional complexity, the success of business schools, or complacency might all have played a part. A simple answer might just be *hysteresis* or inertia. Indeed, this might just be attributable to "status quo bias" or regret avoidance where decision-makers might lose money in a conventional way rather than take risk in an unconventional way that is also related to the unrecoverable or sunk cost fallacy or the Concorde problem (Kahneman and Tversky, 1979; Arkes and Blumer, 1985; Kahneman et al., 1991; Arkes and Ayton, 1999). The strong effect of the pandemic was to cut through the inertia and influence change quickly. Having said that, some of the decisions and approaches to pivot online or a hybrid model might not be as simple to implement successfully in a cost-effective manner, as some educators have imagined.

There are a range of push factors for change, but the challenges for institutions relate to a set of enabling conditions for success, namely the level of trust, value, and legitimacy granted to a given management school by its stakeholders that will influence and impact the school's survival and sustainability (The Economist, 2020).

In succeeding paragraphs, we examine each of the enabling conditions after posing a few initial questions. Can a university degree conducted in a blended, hybrid format be worth the same as an entirely full-time degree? Would the university be able to build high enough reputational capital and hence generate revenue through other sources like executive education if a majority of its flagship MBA or undergraduate degrees are of hybrid or blended form? And how can you create a lifelong community or network of students and faculty when the majority of your degrees are hybrid? Would there be a magic formula involving a creative mix between scalable hybrid modules and complementary in-person modules that would prosper in the current management education space?

TRUST IN INSTITUTIONAL DEGREES

Due to the pandemic, "…More than 1.5 billion children and young people have been affected by school closures worldwide. …" (UNICEF Press Release, 2020) and had to resort to remote learning, if available. Currently, the online education segment forms only about 2% of the $2.2 trillion education market. However, HolonIQ, a global education market intelligence firm, also estimates there is a $74 billion online degree market in 2025 compared to only $36 billion in 2019 pre-pandemic, a cumulative annual growth rate (CAGR) of 12.8% (HolonIQ Research, 2021). These are trends that are becoming even more apparent in management education. There is an increasing demand for professionally oriented education for immediately bankable skills, at the cost of more liberal arts education, even though more academic and business leaders are proposing a creative amalgamation of the two (Harney and Thomas, 2020; Falkenberg and Cannon, 2021). Growth in graduate management education has been highlighted by the mba.com prospective MBA students' survey report in 2021, which re-emphasized the strong increase in demand for business-related graduate programmes globally for managers to upgrade their skills. The interest is quite deep-seated with 70% international students (both men and women) sticking to their plan of studying abroad and embracing face-to-face learning. However, women are more willing to consider online and flexible delivery (AACSB Magazine, 2021).

In sum, the pandemic induced a wide-scale deployment of online learning tools across the spectrum in educational institutions. While this had some temporary disruptive impact on the boundary and separation of home and school, it has also made online learning more widely acceptable even when delivered by schools offering traditionally in-person programmes. In addition, the flexibility has been greatly appreciated particularly by women with young children whose prospects of continuing with a job has been seen to be disproportionately impacted by the pandemic with the so-called "she-cession", making gender disparity even worse (McKinsey Report, 2021). Overall, it seems that trust in degree programmes either full-time or part-time has not abated due to the pandemic; on the contrary, it has opened more avenues for high-quality education and made it more inclusive through the ubiquitous adoption of well-designed technology-based learning.

BRAND VALUE AND COST

From the supply side, private companies like Amazon, LinkedIn, Google, and other tech companies have entered the fray by developing shorter targeted courses and also providing micro-certificates (LinkedIn Covid19 Resources, 2020; AWS Training, 2021). Private and public institutions have also built programmes using partnerships with content providers and platforms like Coursera, Future Learn, and ED-X. These private companies have at least four advantages. First, they are also potential employers and might be able to connect prospective candidates to other employers and to their own network. Second, these companies are aware of the skillsets needed for the job and would be able to design targeted programmes with relevant skills in areas such as in cloud storage, marketing, and other strategic areas. Third, private companies might not have the same cost structure for developing curricula as universities that also have to fund expensive non-commercial research. Hence, private companies can sometimes offer such programmes at a much lower cost as they are unencumbered by costly private-funded academic research. Finally, as highlighted by Professor Scott Galloway, partnerships between elite universities and private companies might be the future of education (Walsh, 2020). There is also a wide brand recognition particularly for those private companies which partner high-quality business schools like Questrom (Boston), Gies (Illinois), and Wharton (Upenn). These would prove attractive for prospective students who might not find enrollment in the top few universities but would nevertheless be able to access a high-quality hybrid MBA programme. Clearly, universities currently developing business and professional programmes need to be fully aware of their edge and competitive advantage in enhancing their hybrid/F2F programmes, without losing their brand value and reputation in the process.

LEGITIMACY, OWNERSHIP, AND FUNDING

Alumni of universities form one of the main sets of stakeholders of a university. However, the pandemic has often precluded current students, faculty, or alumni from engaging in-person with other members of the university. This presents a significant challenge as this directly impacts the interaction and involvement of the student with the alumni community and its ongoing network. Online engagements might be convenient and pleasant, but they do not alone instill a sense of togetherness, either in the short or the long run. In the short run, remote learning and social distancing restrictions during the pandemic has impacted students, particularly in Europe, the United States, and United Kingdom. Students are demanding lower tuition fees (in the United States) or deciding to take gap semesters or study in much lower cost community colleges to transfer credit at a later date when they can attend in-person for major university study. In the long run, those students who missed out on their interaction and networking opportunities might not be willing to make donations to their degree granting universities. Note that universities, particularly private universities in the United States, gain considerable resources from endowment funding (Lerner et al., 2008). Further, their alumni networks might also get weaker, causing further problems such as a reduced likelihood of recruitment of fellow alumni, and less chance of alumni coming back for lifelong and continuing education programmes including executive education. This indeed is a "double whammy" for the university, particularly for small private colleges in the United States whose main source of revenue is through tuition fees. Some of these might have to close doors due to funding shortages as in the case of MacMurray College in Illinois which closed its doors after 174 years of operation (Kennedy, 2020). Business programmes and schools, which thrive on creating interpersonal relationships among their alumni networks and hence increase their influence in the corporate arena, will also suffer greatly from lower government funding and alumni support and, therefore, might also face imminent closure.

THE FUTURE OF MANAGEMENT EDUCATION

With management education facing many challenges, the rankings-based, "winner takes all" mentality might also create impediments for important collaborations with other schools and communities. This competitive mentality must change (Khurana, 2007; Cornuel et al., 2021). Business schools and universities should therefore build on their comparative advantage of connecting with their own regional businesses and schools as well as partnering with other universities in order to create a value proposition that provides a hybrid, stackable solution for many students; in essence, a customized personalized degree that helps each student or alumnus to create a flexible degree that will be valued in the marketplace. Even though examples of collaboration among consortia are quite rare, for example, the Community of European Management Schools (CEMS); CEMS is offering programmes like its highly regarded MSc in Management, which has enabled them to build a network of faculty with expertise, that has generated global collaboration and learning in different parts of the world. It has also cultivated linkages with multi-national businesses to offer hybrid forms of project-based, experiential learning that will enhance students' problem-solving attributes and capabilities.

While we have emphasized the supply side of the suite of offerings of management degrees, the enabling conditions of trust, value, and legitimacy of degrees cannot be overemphasized. Trust in hybrid and online degrees has been amply demonstrated by the surge of demand of online offerings and on the accelerated growth in these programmes (e.g. Illinois, Questrom, Wharton), particularly highlighted by working professionals and the higher propensity of women who favour such programmes. Together with an intrinsic value, there is a "conspicuous consumption" (or luxury good) or Veblen good component present in elite programmes with a positively sloping demand curve for both undergraduate and graduate management degrees (higher price leading to higher demand). However, the value proposition for successful online and hybrid MBA programmes, for example, in Boston, Illinois, Warwick, and Imperial, amply demonstrates a more traditional downward sloping demand curve for management degrees from schools that are not quite as highly ranked as the elite schools yet offer high-quality degrees at competitive prices.

These programmes provide a societal value creation through carefully addressing the difference between the students' "WTP" and the opportunity cost of the suppliers of the content and delivery. This is the true asset value of management education, while non-transferrable, it is a highly portable element of long-term human capital. A final concern is the perceived legitimacy and reputational aspect of hybrid degree programmes in comparison to in-person degree programmes offered by management schools. The experience of successful, adaptive management schools indicates that creative programme design and quality control of both content and intake is key to preserving brand value. In that sense, universities have generally maintained their considerable edge in content creation expertise over disruptive programmes offered by companies like Google and Amazon.

The further value of a management degree from a university emanates from its legitimacy and the portability which certainly appears to be even more in demand in the current climate of uncertainty. This is particularly evident from the report findings of a survey in which, "Among the total responding sample of 1,085 graduate business school programs, 67 percent report that they received more applications for 2020 entry than they did in 2019" (Hazenbush, 2020). COVID-19 has increased the value of management education and reinforced its relevance and impact globally despite wide differences across cultures, contexts, and countries. Deans and administrators have now realized its full potential as a change agent and catalyst for innovation and inclusive growth (Thomas et al., 2013a,b; Thomas et al., 2014; Piketty, 2014; Carlile et al., 2016; Carlile and Thomas, 2020; Piketty, 2019; Thomas and Hedrick-Wong, 2019).

If a prospective investor is exploring the right asset class for portfolio in this uncertain pandemic, volatile world, quoting Nobel Laureate Bob Dylan's famous song about life, "…the answer my friend is blowin' in the wind, the answer is blowin' in the wind…" in a highly customizable quality hybrid of in-person and online instruction in Business School Management programmes.

NOTE

This contributed chapter was accepted for publication in this refereed edited volume on June 17, 2021.

REFERENCES

AACSB Magazine (2021), "High demand for graduate management education," https://www.aacsb.edu/insights/2021/april/high-demand-for-graduate-management-education, May 29, 2021.

Alvarado, G, A. Ghosh and H. Thomas, 2019, "Reputation and Strategic Choices in Business Schools: The Role of Rankings and Accreditations," Working Paper, Singapore Management University, Singapore.

Arkes, H.R. and P. Ayton, (1999), "The sunk-cost and Concorde effects: Are humans less rational than lower animals?" *Psychological Bulletin*, 125, pp. 591–600.

Arkes, H.R. and C. Blumer, (1985), "The psychology of sunk costs," *Organizational Behavior and Human Decision Processes*, 35, pp. 124–140.

Augier, M.E. and J. March, (2011), *The Roots, Rituals and Rhetorics of Change: North American Business Schools After the Second World War*, Stanford, CA: Stanford Business Books.

AWS Training, (2021), "Training and certification: Learn from AWS experts. Advance your skills and knowledge. Build your future in the AWS cloud," https://aws.amazon.com/training/, May 29, 2021.

Bloomberg News, (2021), "Central banks to pour money into economy despite sharp rebound," https://www.bloomberg.com/news/articles/2021-04-19/robust-rebound-won-t-augur-end-to-stimulus-central-bank-guide, May 29, 2021.

Brandenburger, A.M. and H.W. Stuart Jr., (1996), "Value-based business strategy," *Journal of Economics and Management Strategy*, 5(1), pp. 5–24.

Carlile, P.R., S.H. Davidson, K.W. Freeman, H. Thomas and N. Venkatraman, (2016), *Re-imagining Business Education: Insights and Actions from the Business Education Jam*, Bingley: Emerald Publishing.

CARES Act, (2020), "CARES Act: Higher education emergency relief fund," https://www2.ed.gov/about/offices/list/ope/caresact.html, May 29, 2021.

Carlile, P.R. and H. Thomas, (2020), "How to develop collaborative projects that drive innovation," Global Focus, 14(2), pp. 39–43.

Cassim, Z., B. Handjiski, J. Schubert, and Y. Zouaoui, (2020), "The $10 trillion rescue: How governments can deliver impact," McKinsey & Company Report, https://www.mckinsey.com/~/media/McKinsey/Industries/Public%20Sector/Our%20Insights/The%2010%20trillion%20dollar%20rescue%20How%20governments%20can%20deliver%20impact/The-10-trillion-dollar-rescue-How-governments-can-deliver-impact-vF.pdf, May 29, 2021.

Cattani, G., J.F. Porac and H. Thomas, (2017), "Categories and competition," Strategic Management Journal, 38(1), pp. 64–92.

Cornuel, E., H. Thomas and M. Wood, (2021), "Looking back and thinking forward," *Global Focus*, 15th Anniversary Issue, Brussels, Belgium: EFMD Publications.

Coronavirus Job Retention Scheme, (2020), "Claim for wages through the Coronavirus Job Retention Scheme," https://www.gov.uk/guidance/claim-for-wages-through-the-coronavirus-job-retention-scheme, May 29, 2021.

El-Erian, M., (2021), "When is stimulus too much for markets?" https://www.ft.com/content/6254971a-96dd-41a9-a037-acf3ffa6275b, May 29, 2021.

Falkenberg, L. and M.E. Cannon, (2021), "To 'future proof' universities, leaders have to engage faculty to make tough decisions," The Conversation, https://theconversation.com/to-future-proof-universities-leaders-have-to-engage-faculty-to-make-tough-decisions-155285?_cldee=YXVVyb2JpbmRvQHNttd-

S51ZHUuc2c%3d&recipientid=lead-018b4f081c89e91180f-4000d3a01cfd3-8ad63666fe93464b94507d7ad72da465&utm_source=ClickDimensions&utm_medium=email&utm_campaign=LINK&esid=3b3ab707-45a1-eb11-810f-000d3a01cfd3, May 29, 2021.

Frey, C.B. and M.A. Osbourne, (2017), "The future of employment: How susceptible are jobs to computerisation?" *Technological Forecasting and Social Change*, 114, pp. 254–280.

Ghoshal, S., (2005), "Bad management theories are destroying good management practices," *Academy of Management Learning and Education*, 4(1), pp. 75–91.

Gordon, R.A. and J.E. Howell, (1959), *Higher Education for Business*, New York: Columbia University Press.

Harney, S. and H. Thomas, (2020), *The Liberal Arts and Management Education: A Global Agenda for Change*, Cambridge: Cambridge University Press.

Hazenbush, M., (2020), "MBA applications spiked in 2020—What's that mean for 2021?" https://www.mba.com/information-and-news/research-and-data/mba-applications-spike-2020-implications-for-2021, May 31, 2021.

HolonIQ Research, (2021), "$74B online degree market in 2025, up from $36B in 2019," https://www.holoniq.com/notes/74b-online-degree-market-in-2025-up-from-36b-in-2019/, May 29, 2021.

Kahneman, D., J.L. Knetsch and R.H. Thaler, (1991), "Anomalies: The endowment effect, loss aversion, and status quo bias," *The Journal of Economic Perspectives*, 5(1), pp. 193–206.

Kahneman, D. and A. Tversky, (1979), "Prospect theory: An analysis of decisions under risk," *Econometrica*, 47, pp. 263–291.

Kandri, S.-E., (2020), "How COVID-19 is driving a long-overdue revolution in education," https://www.weforum.org/agenda/2020/05/how-covid-19-is-sparking-a-revolution-in-higher-education, May 29, 2021.

Kennedy, M., (2020), "MacMurray college is closing after 174 years," https://www.asumag.com/facilities-management/article/21128166/macmurray-college-is-closing-after-174-years, May 29, 2021.

Khurana, R., (2007), *From Higher Aims to Hired Hands: The Social Transformation of American Business Schools and the Unfulfilled Promise of Management as a Profession, Princeton*, NJ: Princeton University Press.

Kong, L. and S. Patra, (2022), "Universities in and beyond a pandemic," In Ghosh, Haldar and Bhaumik, Edited, *Managing Complexity and Covid-19: Life, Liberty, or the Pursuit of Happiness*, Routledge, pp. 20–35.

Lerner, J., A. Schoar and J. Wang, (2008), "Secrets of the academy: The drivers of university endowment success," *Journal of Economic Perspectives*, 22(3), pp. 207–222.

LinkedIn COVID-19 Resources, (2020), "8 learning paths to help you develop your skills — No matter what role or industry you're in," https://about.linkedin.com/coronavirus-resource-hub/online-courses, May 29, 2021.

MBA CSEA Report, (2020), "2020 MBA CSEA fall recruiting trend survey," https://www.mbacsea.org/Files/Fall%202020%20Recruiting%20Trends%20Survey%20Summary%20Report.pdf, May 29, 2021.

McGee, J. and H. Thomas, (1986), "Strategic groups: Theory, research and taxonomy." *Strategic Management Journal*, 7(2), pp. 141–160.

McKinsey Report, (2021), "Seven charts that show COVID-19's impact on women's employment," https://www.mckinsey.com/featured-insights/diversity-and-inclusion/seven-charts-that-show-covid-19s-impact-on-womens-employment, May 29, 2021.

Paycheck Protection Program, (2020), "Paycheck protection program," https://www.sba.gov/funding-programs/loans/covid-19-relief-options/pay-check-protection-program, May 29, 2020.

Peters, K., R.R. Smith and H. Thomas, (2018), *The Business of Business Schools*, Bingley: Emerald Publishing.

Pfeffer, J. and C.T. Fong, (2004), "The business school business – Some lessons from the U.S. experience," *Journal of Management Studies*, 41(8), pp. 1501–1520.

Piketty, T., (2014), *Capital in the Twenty-First Century*, Cambridge, MA: Belknap Press.

Piketty, T., (2019), *Capital and Ideology*, (Translated by Arthur Goldhammer), Cambridge, MA: Harvard University Press.

Policano, A., (2005), "What price rankings?" *BizEd*, September-October, Tampa, FL: AACSB Publications

Ranasinghe, D. and S. Rao, (2020), "Central banks have thrown many tools at coronavirus. What do they have left?" https://www.reuters.com/article/us-health-coronavirus-cenbank-graphic-idUSKBN23W2D9, May 29, 2021.

Schoemaker, P.J.H., (2008), "The future challenges of business: Re-thinking management education," *California Management Review*, 50(3), pp. 119–139.

Simonson, I. and A. Drolet, "Anchoring effects on consumers' willingness-to-pay and willingness-to-accept," (2003), Research Paper No. 1787, Graduate School of Business, Stanford University, USA.

Starkey, K and H. Thomas, (2019), "The future of business schools: Shut them down or broaden our horizons," *Global Focus*, 13(2), pp. 44–49.

Taras, V., G. Shah, M. Gunkel, and E. Tavoletti, (2020), "Graduates of elite universities get paid more. Do they perform better?" *Harvard Business Review*, https://hbr.org/2020/09/graduates-of-elite-universities-get-paid-more-do-they-perform-better, May 29, 2021.

The Economist, 2009, "It's expensive, so it must be good," https://www.economist.com/free-exchange/2009/09/02/its-expensive-so-it-must-be-good, May 29, 2021.

The Economist, 2020, ""Some were struggling to attract students and running pretty big deficits"—universities and covid-19," https://www.economist.com/podcasts/2020/05/05/some-were-struggling-to-attract-students-and-running-pretty-big-deficits-universities-and-covid-19, May 29, 2021.

Thomas, H. and Y. Hedrick-Wong, (2019), *Inclusive Growth: The Global Challenges of Social Inequality and Financial Inclusion*, Bingley: Emerald Publishing.

Thomas, H., M. Lee, L. Thomas and A. Wilson, (2013a), *Securing the Future of Management Education*. Bingley: Emerald Publishing.

Thomas, H., P. Lorange and J. Sheth, (2014), *The Business School in the 21st Century: Emergent Challenges and New Business Models*, Cambridge: Cambridge University Press.

Thomas, H., L. Thomas and A. Wilson, (2013b), *Promises Fulfilled and Unfulfilled in Management Education*, Bingley: Emerald Publishing.

UNICEF Press Release, (2020), "Children at increased risk of harm online during global COVID-19 pandemic," https://www.unicef.org/press-releases/children-increased-risk-harm-online-during-global-covid-19-pandemic, May 29, 2021.

Veblen, T., (1899), *The Theory of the Leisure Class; an Economic Study of Institutions*, New York: Dover Editions.

Walsh, J.D., (2020), "HIGHER EDUCATION: The coming disruption Scott Galloway predicts a handful of elite cyborg universities will soon monopolize higher education," https://nymag.com/intelligencer/2020/05/scott-galloway-future-of-college.html, May 29, 2021.

Wolf, M., (2021), "The return of the inflation spectre," https://www.ft.com/content/6cfb36ca-d3ce-4dd3-b70d-eecc332ba1df, May 29, 2021.

4

ECONOMICS BIFURCATIONS AND ASYMMETRIES

Taimur Baig

WHEN THE REACTION CAME TOO LATE

As the pandemic spread from China to Europe and then to the rest of the world in early 2020, there was initial reluctance among those in charge of policy response to recognize the obvious fact that infectious diseases know no borders. To be fair, recent episodes like SARS in 2003, may have played a role in the relatively sluggish response. During that pandemic, once the outbreak spread, a policy of detection was enforced through temperature and symptoms checking, which proved to be highly successful in isolating the carriers of the virus. The initial view with COVID-19 was that setting up temperature checking stations and tracking additional symptoms would suffice.

Why were forecasters and market participants oblivious of the gravity of the situation? Even if it was not possible to gauge the impending global outbreak, it was well known that China had imposed stringent restrictions on mobility by the third week of January. The substantial role that China plays in the global supply chain, and the reliance of commodity markets and goods exporters on Chinese demand, have been evident for many years, so why was the rapidly worsening situation in China not worrying economists and financial markets?

Looking back on those pivotal days in early 2020, when it took global markets nearly a month after China's lockdown to appreciate the global implications of the outbreak, with the S&P 500 hitting a record

DOI: 10.4324/9781003218807-5

high on February 18, a few points are now clear. First, neither epidemiologists nor market participants appreciated the virulence of the novel coronavirus, especially the route of asymptomatic infection. This had never happened before, and hence there was simply no way to prepare for the extent of the impending outbreak. Second, even if there was some appreciation of the lockdown unfolding in China, the view remained that this would be temporary, with only modest impact on production, shipping, and transportation. Boeing's stock price is instructive in this context, which remained unaffected through the middle of February despite growing risks to global travel.

By the third week of February, the depth of the unfolding crisis began to dawn, and markets not just caught up, they corrected ahead of widespread public health responses. Even before Italy went into lockdown on March 8/9, global markets had declined by just about the most it would during this crisis. Economists also joined in, and substantial downward revision to global growth began in earnest as it became obvious that the whole world was about to experience severe restrictions to mobility, with highly uncertain but likely devastating impact on lives forthcoming.

This stock-taking of the first two months of the pandemic is important as it illustrates the inadequate forecasting and *Nowcasting* tools available in economics and finance when it comes to assessing tail events like a pandemic. This shortcoming has troubled industry professionals in the past as well, for instance, in 2008/09, the complex global inter-linkage and contagion implications of the US subprime market was not captured by Wall Street or professional forecasters until it was too late. In this instance, the fault lies not just with those in economics and finance; after all, they have no choice but to take cues on pandemic risks from public health officials. Looking forward, further appreciation of tail risks and reforming public health response systems that are nimble and adoptable to evolving risks would be an imperative.

A DOUBLE WHAMMY AND A SPECTACULAR REBOUND

The 1970s oil shock came from the supply side. The 2008 crisis began with credit rationing which morphed into a profound demand shock. The COVID pandemic combined the worst of both crises.

On the demand side, in a matter of days, thriving industries in the areas of travel, tourism, in-person retail, dining, beauty, and fitness had come to a standstill. For a while, even agriculture, food processing, manufacturing, and construction were severely disrupted. Resulting loss of jobs and income were immediate. Faced with such a dramatic development and major uncertainties about their lives and livelihood, consumer demand became extremely cautious, withholding consumption and pushing up saving rates.

On the supply side, production was disrupted as infections spread through assembly lines, meat processing plants, and even farms. Shortages of essentials manifested almost immediately, with empty store shelves becoming a ubiquitous feature of the pandemic's fallout. Besides plant closures, shipping lanes and ports also faced closures, disrupting the availability of parts. Spooked by the dismal demand outlook, manufacturers scaled back production, perpetuating the entire situation.

Forecasters may have been playing catch-up, but by mid-March the outlook was clear—a recession of global proportions was unfolding, with the downside even greater than that experienced during the 2008/09 financial crisis. In April, the International Monetary Fund (IMF) forecasted 3% contraction in global growth for the year, far worse than the outcome in 2008/09. What was even more dramatic was that the forecast represented a 6 percent point swing in the outlook, as the IMF was expecting around 3% global growth in January 2020.

As the pandemic deepened in Europe and the United States, forecasts were revised down further in mid-June, but by this time forecasters were falling behind the underlying developments, in the other direction. The IMF's June forecast of nearly minus 5% global growth for the year proved to be too pessimistic, and long before actual data could settle the case, global markets roared back from May onwards. While policymakers and forecasters may have been in highly uncertain times, financial markets were already latching onto the winners in the pandemic economy, pushing up equity prices along the way.

Who were the economic winners? Those who benefitted from the disruption in activities ranged from delivery services to e-commerce, from producers of communication devices to electronic content. If there was a service or good suited for work from home, its value, and the value of the company that produced it, soared. It also became apparent by then that global technology infrastructure was resilient enough to stand up to the crisis-driven spike in usage.

The other major factor driving a revival in global market sentiment was of course the policy response. Putting on their crisis-fighting hats, major central banks cut interest rates down to their floor, injected record quantities of liquidity by purchasing bonds worth hundreds of billions of dollars, opened lending windows to a wide range of borrowers, and offered swap lines to other central banks to prevent panic and runs. Fiscal authorities shed their conservative garbs, allowing their fiscal deficits to widen sharply, which were measured in trillions of dollars, passing wide-ranging spending and cash transfer programmes to support businesses and households.

All these helped bond and stock prices to soar, property markets to rebound, the dread of deflation to disappear, and liquidity to turn ample. By the end of 2020, market-based activities had helped many financial institutions to profit handsomely, capital markets were replete with large-scale transactions, government bond and corporate credit spreads narrowed to pre-pandemic levels, and the phrase "reflation trade" was in wide use. Economic activities rebounded and unemployment rate began to decline sharply. With vaccinations taking off and stimulus-driven demand gaining strength, the world's two largest economies, China and the United States, looked forward to 2021, when they could make up for the lost output from the year of the pandemic.

MASKED BY THE REBOUND

The spectacular turnaround in asset prices and financial profits, along with stimulus-supported rebound in demand worldwide, mask a few harsh realities. A crisis of this magnitude causes deep scarring that no amount of stock market rebound can smooth over. From accelerated disruption to women in the workplace, from the accentuated digital divide to the paucity of social safety nets, the pandemic has highlighted many bifurcations, within and between societies.

With a few exceptions, most economies will take years to make up for the lost output of 2020, and in many cases the event would mark a permanent downshift in trend output level. This may appear surprising, as the shock seems to dissipate with a successful public health response. But a deeper examination of the crisis reveals a peculiar nature of the recovery and the scarring that will most likely come with it.

The rebound from the depths of the crisis has been uneven across the board. Sectors that contribute to remote work, distance learning, digital streaming, and all other manner of electronics have thrived, while many traditional sectors that focused on human interaction have faded. Their disruption was merely accelerated by the pandemic, whose sunset was looming in any case.

As disruptions are accelerated, the path out of the crisis becomes naturally bifurcated or k-shaped. Some sectors come out strongly, while some hobble, perhaps terminally. This has a knock-on impact on the labour market, as those with skills suitable for the sunset sectors find their human capital rapidly eroded in the post-pandemic world.

These bifurcations are vividly visible at the micro level. Consider the move toward work from home, a shift that has its positives. It allows workers to spend less time commuting, which is good for their health, and expands the time available for family and recreation. It also reduces inefficiencies related to travels for meetings, nudges workers to improve their skills and productivity by using technology, and lowers emission due to the reduction in work-related travel. But it is not all positive. Remote working reduces demand for city living, which in turn reduces demand for city services. At first glance, this might seem to be merely a transitional cost, as the decrease in demand from urban services ought to be made up by a concomitant rise in suburban demand. But, in fact, the transition leads to permanent, non-offsetting losses. Some services, fine dining or art galleries, for example, are only viable in a dense, high-volume environment; they become unviable in a diffused setting. Such services are often the standard-setter for trends and innovative practices. A society where the cities have hollowed out will likely be characterized by a viable but non-dynamic sprawl of suburbs. As workers spend less time in cities, avenues for live exchange of ideas, serendipitous encounters that lead to opportunities and network building, become rarer, which leaves everyone worse off.

With schools shut down for an extended period, families had to make difficult adjustments, and in numerous instances women have had to incur most of the costs. They have often had to be the ones to give up their jobs to take care of stay-at-home children, and when the kids went back to school, have had to grapple with already-eroded human capital and an altered employment landscape. Also, women are disproportionally represented in food services, retail, and education, sectors that have been most affected by the pandemic. Women also tend to lose their access to savings and financial capital during periods of economic distress, and evidence from both emerging and developed markets suggest the same was the case during the COVID pandemic.

Digital divide is often thought of in the context of developing versus developed economies, but that is only part of the picture. In developed countries with inadequate provisions for public housing for the poor, the digital divide is accentuated among the homeless. This is particularly the case in the United States, where millions of school-going children lack permanent addresses, rendering remote schooling from "home" somewhat unfeasible. Thus, the pandemic created a commonality of experience among the vulnerable, across societies.

Without exception, a lockdown affects the poor disproportionally, with livelihoods interrupted, insufficient financial buffers, inadequate access to digital infrastructure, and typically cramped living conditions. With respect to housing, the urban poor, living in congested environments, are not only unable to perform remote tasks adequately, their vulnerability to infection is also heightened given the impossibility of social distancing.

Adopting to accelerated disruption, budgeting at a time of financial insecurity and uncertainty, striking a balance between spending, saving, and investing are particularly burdensome for the poor, who have neither the time nor the education to make the requisite, rapid adjustments. These factors make for deep transitional costs and increasing likelihood of long-term unemployment or underemployment.

Vulnerabilities of women, minorities, and the poor can be addressed by social safety net measures, both temporary and permanent. Among temporary measures, economists favour paycheck supplements for all through direct cash transfers, extension and augmentation of unemployment benefits, incentives for companies to not lay off staff, and support for jobs training for those laid off. On the permanent side, childcare benefits, universal health insurance, support for job creation in emerging industries, funding public pension, and education grants are likely to help build better quality human capital and reduce insecurity. These measures not only help mitigate the inequities in the society but also are critical in reducing the amplitude of the business cycle. The economy's ability to absorb shocks improve through a well-targeted social safety net and the seeds for sustainable growth in the future are sown.

Labour market measures are critical due to the fundamental asymmetry embedded in crises. A lockdown causes unemployment to spike immediately, but the easing of lockdowns does not cause employment to jump in a similar manner. Going back to the pre-crisis level of 3.5% rate of unemployment, reached in February 2020, will take years to retrace, if at all. Beyond the hard work needed to push down unemployment, policymakers will have to also grapple with a shrinking labour force, caused by skill mismatches discouraging some workers.

CLIMATE CHANGE AGENDA: AT RISK OR A PANACEA?

The cost of dealing with this crisis has already manifested in large increases in fiscal deficits and debt. Countries as disparate as the United States, India, and Singapore saw their public sector debt/GDP ratios jump by 11–25% in 2020, with more expansion likely in the near term.

Will the pandemic leave policymakers, corporations, and civil societies so exhausted from the ordeal that there will be a loss of interest in other matters of importance? Will we be so impoverished that our generosity to set aside resources toward important causes will dissipate, and governments will loath spending in priority areas?

In recent years, there has been a sizeable shift toward taking actions to fight climate change, reduce poverty, improve livelihood (health, education, quality of work), and the social imperative of companies (including stakeholder accountability). While much more remains to be done, there has been an increase in resources devoted to dealing with these issues, and there has been a discernible shift in public perception toward living in a society that is more just, and a world that is more sustainable.

It is easy to worry that post-pandemic priorities will shift to issues closer to the pocketbook, like restoring jobs and boosting asset markets. But this cynicism is most likely misplaced.

During the lockdown months of 2020, social media was rife with photos of bright blue skies in cities previously overcast with pollution, and dark canals and rivers turning clear and transparent. Meanwhile, affliction from breathing high particulate air fell dramatically. Nature's ability to heal and rebound has seldom been so starkly demonstrated. As the terrible pandemic ends, will we simply go back to business as usual, or will we reach out to policy measures and technological solutions that allow us to hold on to what has been regained in recent months?

Beyond responding to the romanticism of blue skies and fresh air, policymakers have a harder truth to deal with in the post-pandemic world. To propel their economies forward, national authorities will have to take into account long-lasting downshift in the demand for travel, tourism, dining out, sports events, and concerts. The imperative to find a major engine of growth to offset a possible depression is considerable.

With key engines of growth sputtering, what better way to galvanize public sentiments and direct a big chunk of the declared support measures to climate change and better societal outcomes? A win–win solution would be to divert investments and job creation efforts in the renewable energy industry, green infrastructure, low or zero emission transportation, education, and health. This ought to be coupled with policy measures to reduce income distortions and disparity, and hence, increase wealth transfers toward a more humane and equitable society. In short, ensuring a "just transition."

Dealing with a crisis like this underscores the need for well-targeted social safety nets, comprehensive public health provisions, and national stockpiles of products to deal with extreme events. It also reminds us that there are many shocks in which we are all in together. Acute inequality makes the society inherently unstable as the frustration and despair of the deprived make for a demotivated and socially volatile population. Similarly, a country with a weak public health system or a world with inadequate response to rising sea levels will remain fragile.

How much are developing countries spending on dealing with tuberculosis, HIV/AIDS, and malaria? Estimates suggest marked increases in the past decade, but still falling far short of what is needed. Among the countries with the most pressing needs, there is still over-reliance on donor funding. The COVID-19 crisis ought to galvanize support for more own-source financing for such public health needs. Chastened by the pandemic, the public and policy-makers will surely become more serious about sustainable development goals, one of which aims to "ensure healthy lives and promote well-being for all ages."

This crisis has revealed many misplaced priorities. Trillions go toward building and maintaining weapons of mass destruction, but billions are cut from public health provisions. Businesses worry about the flow of credit and the risk of default, but do not fully recognize the impact climate change will have on their operations and product demand. We worry about upgrading to newer cars and phones but ignore basic practices of hygiene and sustainability. Behind such behaviour runs the undercurrent that third world health, climate change, and rare pandemics are too big and too macro, and they must be someone else's problem. Social scientists agonize over ways to bring public attention to these critically important but regularly neglected matters. The enabling window for action is, however, opening as we live, learn, and empathize through this global cataclysm.

NOTE

This contributed chapter was accepted for publication in this refereed edited volume on July 1, 2021.

5

TAMING THE PANDEMIC BY DOING THE MUNDANE

*Satarupa Bhattacharjee, Shuting Liao,
Debashis Paul, and Sanjay Chaudhuri*

INTRODUCTION

The ongoing COVID-19 pandemic has posed one of the greatest challenges to humanity in recent times. The human cost in terms of lives lost to the pandemic has been staggering, as well as the economic cost for mitigation. Even though arrival of effective vaccines in late 2020 has raised hopes substantially, in terms of finally bringing an end to the pandemic, inadequate vaccine availability coupled with distribution issues, have contributed to repeated surges at a global level. All of these have given rise to debates about the relative effectiveness of measures such as increased diagnostic testing and vaccination coupled with intervention measures. The latter includes restricting the social mobility by imposing lockdowns and strict masking mandates. The economic impact of various measures undertaken by governments bring about the unfortunate choice between saving lives versus preserving collective economic well-being (see, e.g., Prem et al., 2020; Soltesz et al., 2020; Susskind and Vines, 2020; Bubar et al., 2021; Cirakli et al., 2021; Mbwogge, 2021). Prioritizing the latter resulted in a few countries initially attempting to achieve "herd immunity" through unfettered propagation of virus in the community, typically with disastrous consequences for public health, and at no small cost to the economy (Brett and Rohani, 2020; Kwok et al., 2020; Randolph and Barreiro, 2020).

DOI: 10.4324/9781003218807-6

These facts obviate the paramount importance of bringing all the elements—epidemiological, interventionist, and economic— together in forming a policy decision, at a regional or national level. In addition, for an effective policy, it is necessary to also consider factors like the intrinsic capacity of the healthcare system and differential levels of vulnerability to the disease, among different segments of the population. Existing literature on the COVID pandemic mostly ignore the question of appropriate policy decisions, in terms of adopting specific intervention measures, while incorporating the different contributing factors as well as the economic impact.

The focus of this study is to find a policy in the form of an optimal degree of social distancing, typically executed through a combination of lockdown and physical distancing. This optimal decision is obtained by minimizing a cost function, aggregated over a fixed time horizon that aims to limit total mortality and severe illness, consistent with the ultimate objective of most vaccine development (also see Ghosh, 2022; Part II in this volume), while also being responsive to the economic costs of lockdown, under existing constraints in terms of the capacity of the healthcare system. We also investigate the impact of various rates of testing and vaccination.

In order to achieve this, we introduce a discrete-time deterministic dynamic model for the disease dynamics on a network, the nodes of which represent different geographical entities, or population segments, with differential levels of vulnerability to the disease. The proposed compartmental model is akin to SIR (Susceptible-Infected-Recovered) or SEIR (Susceptible-Exposed-Infectious-Removed) models popularly used in modelling the pandemic (see, e.g., Giordano et al., 2020; Tolles and Luong, 2020). However, it incorporates the effects of migration (Kucharski et al., 2020) as well as social distancing on the dynamics (Badr et al., 2020). Moreover, the model integrates the effect of testing and quarantining people, as well as vaccination. Specific rate parameters in the model are chosen from the analyses of COVID-19 data in the United States (see Bhattacharjee et al., 2021). Therefore, the model is expected to be a realistic emulator of this complex epidemiological process. The cost function for optimization, admittedly limited in its scope, is set as a sum of the loss of economic output resulting from deaths of COVID-19, and that from the spells of lockdown.

We perform a comprehensive set of simulations that idealize different scenarios and compare the corresponding optimal policy choices and their human and economic costs. The main conclusion of our analyses is that there is no stand–alone measure that can bring the pandemic under control within a reasonable time frame. Rather, it is necessary to combine a set of policy measures to limit the human and economic costs to a low level. Even then, there may be a need for multiple rounds of lockdown to dampen the surges in infection. Moreover, even with vaccination, natural "herd immunity" is not a practical policy option even from an economic point of view if one carefully factors in the true economic costs. These conclusions are generally consistent with the experience across the world. Therefore, it is expected that the proposed framework can act as a useful workbench for health policy options at local or regional levels in addressing the enormous challenges posed by the pandemic.

MECHANISTIC MODEL FOR A VIRAL EPIDEMIC

Compartments of the System

We propose a network-based multi-compartmental model to mimic the progression of a pandemic in terms of various observable and partially or totally unobservable compartments. We consider a network of N nodes, each representing a population centre (e.g. country) with different nodes possibly having different levels of vulnerability to the disease. The model incorporates migration among the nodes.

We use t to denote time (in days), and k to denote nodes. For node k, D_{kt} denotes the number of deaths up to time t. Notations for other compartments are similar. The epidemic dynamics is assumed to be memoryless, meaning that the compartment transition rates are independent of the duration of stay in a particular compartment. Definitions of the compartments and the epidemiological and intervention parameters are given in Table 5.1. More detailed definitions and underlying model assumptions are given in Section 1 of the Supplementary material (www.routledge.com/9781032115160).

Table 5.1 Definition of the compartments and the epidemiological and intervention parameters. More details can be found in the Supplement (www.routledge.com/9781032115160).

Compartments	Parameters	
Unobservable	Epidemiological: (transition rates)	Intervention
S: susceptible J: infected but asymptomatic G: uninfected individuals quarantined due to a false-positive test	γ_k: asymptomatic to symptomatic α_k: asymptomatic to recovered ζ_k: recovery from symptomatic without hospitalization	ω_{jk}: daily rate of migration from node j to k $\omega_{jk}: e\big(\beta_{0k} + \beta_{1k}\Delta D_{jt}\big)\big/\big\{1 + e\big(\beta_{0k} + \beta_{1k}\Delta D_{jt}\big)\big\}$
Observable	ξ_{kpk}: symptomatic to hospitaliza- tion to recovered δ_k: mortality rate ι_c: basic infection coefficient	I_{kt}: Infection rate at node k at time t
I: symptomatic individuals D: death IV: vaccinated H: hospitalized Q: quarantined T: tested		$I_{kt}: \iota_{c\mu kt}J_{kt}/(S_{kt} + J_{kt} + R_{kt} + IV_{kt})$ $\mu_{kt}: \mu_{kk2kt}$ μ_k: the number of people an average individual in node k meets on a day in the absence of any restrictions
Partially observable	Clinical	K_{kt}: the fraction of people allowed outside within node k, at time t
R: recovered	$\phi_{kt}: \psi_{FTkt}/(S_{kt} + J_{kt})$ $\tau_{kt}: \psi_{TTkt}/(S_{kt} + J_{kt})$ ψ_F: true-positive rate of test ψ_T: false-positive rate of the test v_k: rate of vaccination at the kth node	

DESCRIPTION OF THE DYNAMICS

The evolution of the pandemic is expressed mechanistically through equations (1)–(9). They capture the mean daily change in the values of the compartments. A graphical representation of the proposed disease propagation model is presented in Figure 5.1.

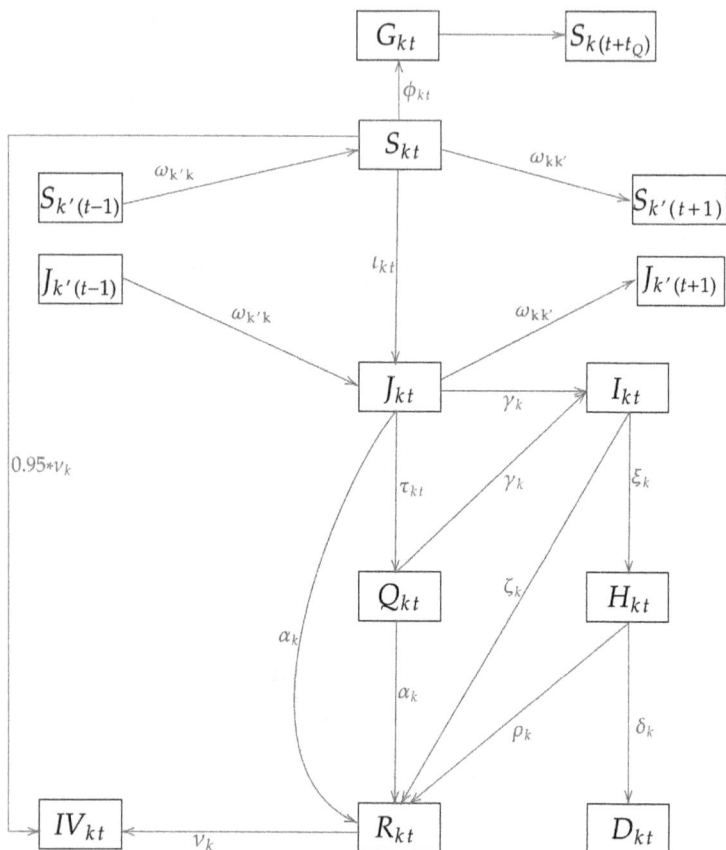

Figure 5.1 Diagram showing the different stages of the propagation of the pandemic for the kth node at time t

A key model assumption is that all infected individuals are initially asymptomatic, after which they either start to show symptoms, get tested and quarantined, or recover directly. The disease spreads through the asymptomatic but infected individuals. We assume that uninfected individuals, falsely caught in the quarantine net, join the susceptible population after t_Q days of self-isolation. Both susceptible (S) and recovered (R) groups are vaccinated, with the vaccination efficacy assumed to be 95% and 100% for these groups, respectively. Once vaccinated the individuals play no further role in the progression of the epidemic. Our model ignores birth and deaths due to other causes (Ivorra et al., 2020). Migration (with time-dependent rate) is only allowed between the susceptible and asymptomatic populations of the nodes.

$$\Delta S_{kt} = \sum_{j:j\neq k} w_{jk} S_{jt} - \sum_{j:j\neq k} w_{kj} S_{kt} - \left(\iota_{kt} + \varphi_{kt} + 0.95 v k\right) S_{kt} + G_{k\left(t - t_Q\right)}, \quad (5.1)$$

$$\Delta J_{kt} = \sum_{j:j\neq k} w_{jk} J_{jt} - \sum_{j:j\neq k} w_{kj} J_{kt} - \left(\tau kt + \gamma k + \alpha k\right) J_{kt} + \iota_{kt} S_{kt}, \quad (5.2)$$

$$\Delta G_{kt} = \varphi_{kt} S_{kt} - G_{k(t-t_Q)}, \quad (5.3)$$

$$\Delta I_{kt} = \gamma k \left(J_{kt} + Q_{kt}\right) - \left(\zeta_k + \xi_k\right) I_{kt}, \quad (5.4)$$

$$\Delta Q_{kt} = \tau kt J_{kt} - \left(\gamma k + \alpha_k\right) Q_{kt}, \quad (5.5)$$

$$\Delta H_{kt} = \xi_k I_{kt} - \left(\rho k + \delta_k\right) H_{kt}, \quad (5.6)$$

$$\Delta R_{kt} = \alpha_k \left(J_{kt} + Q_{kt}\right) + \zeta_k I_{kt} + \rho_k H_{kt} - v_k R_{kt}, \quad (5.7)$$

$$\Delta IV_{kt} = 0.95 v_k S_{kt} + v_k R_{kt}, \quad (5.8)$$

$$\Delta D_{kt} = \delta_k H_{kt}. \quad (5.9)$$

Intervention through Optimal Lockdown

Other than vaccination, imposition of a lockdown with various severity has been useful in controlling the spread of the pandemic. Lockdowns undeniably reduce death and hospitalization but may incur significant socio-economic costs. The mass migration of workers in India, during the nationwide lockdown in 2020, and the staggering number of deaths in the second wave in 2021, when lockdowns were localized and mostly delayed, have abundantly displayed the degree of humanitarian crises associated with unplanned lockdowns. A cost-balanced strategy for imposing lockdowns should therefore be quite beneficial.

We device an optimal lockdown strategy by combining two considerations. A lockdown is imposed whenever either the node-specific hospitalization rate exceeds a certain threshold η_{kt}, or the number of symptomatic people exceed a certain fixed lower bound. The severity of the lockdown is controlled by the social distancing parameter κ_{kt} (between 0 and 1, with 0 indicating complete lockdown). The optimal choice of (η_{kt}, κ_{kt}) ensures that at all times and at all nodes, the hospital capacity (assumed 0.5% of the nodal population) is never exceeded. This is achieved by solving the constrained optimization problem:

$$
\begin{cases}
\left(\widehat{k}_{kt}, \widehat{\eta}_{kt}\right) = \underset{(k_{kt}, \eta_{kt})}{\operatorname{argmin}} \, \Phi\left(k_{kt}, \eta_{kt}\right) \text{ such that } 0 \leq k_{kt}, \eta_{kt} \leq 1, \text{ and} \\
\text{the proportion of hospitalised stays below 0.005, for all } k \text{ and } t.
\end{cases}
$$

(5.10)

The objective function $\Phi(\kappa_{kt}, \eta_{kt})$ balances the economic cost of death with that of the cost of lockdown. In particular, we define:

$$
\Phi\left(k_{kt}, \eta_{kt}\right) = \frac{1}{W} \times \frac{\sum_{k=1}^{N} D_{kT}\left(k_{kt}, \eta_{kt}\right)}{\sum_{k=1}^{N} S_{k1}} + \frac{\sum_{k=1}^{N} \sum_{t=1}^{T} C_{kt}\left(k_{kt}, \eta_{kt}\right)}{\sum_{k=1}^{N} S_{k1}} \quad (5.11)
$$

The economic cost of the lockdown is represented by the term:

$$
C_{kt}\left(k_{kt}, \eta_{kt}\right) = \begin{cases}
\dfrac{\left(1 - k_{kt}\right)\left(S_{kt} + J_{kt} + R_{kt} + IV_{kt}\right)}{30 \times 365} \\
0
\end{cases} \quad (5.12)
$$

This cost function takes into account the economic cost borne by those among the susceptible, asymptomatic, recovered, and immunized people whose work opportunities are lost during lockdown periods. On day t at node k, the fraction among these groups losing their job opportunities is $(1 - \kappa_{kt})$. The factor 365 in the denominator signifies the fact that the economic cost is measured in terms of loss of per capita annualized GDP, while the factor 30 is the (assumed) expected number of additional years a person may live, if he/she does not succumb to the disease. That is, effectively, we equate each death to a loss of 30 years of per capita GDP. The positive factor W in (11) incorporates the relative importance of death vis-à-vis the economic cost of lockdown.

CASE STUDIES

To explore the effects of testing and vaccination, we perform a simulation study by generating the compartmental trajectories from the proposed model. The analyses are carried out over a time horizon of $T = 400$ days, using the epidemiological parameters given in Table 5.2.

Table 5.2 The epidemic parameters for the nodes in the case studies

Epidemic parameter	ι_c	γ	α	ζ	ξ	ρ	δ
Vulnerable node	0.1	0.03	0.005	0.05	0.2	0.07	0.03
Robust node	0.1	0.01	0.02	0.1	0.1	0.15	0.03

Table 5.3 Initial value (on day t = 1) of the number of susceptible S_{k1} and asymptomatic but infected people J_{k1} for each node k

Node k	1	2	3	4	5	6	7	8	9	10
S_{k1}	450,000	449,900	450,000	350,000	350,000	350,000	350,000	350,000	250,000	250,000
J_{k1}	0	100	0	0	0	0	0	0	0	0
Tests, T_{k1}	1,000	1,000	1,000	1,000	1,000	500	500	500	500	500
μ_k	3	3	3	3	3	5	5	5	5	5

Table 5.4 Vaccination rates and daily testing capacities under different scenarios considered in the six cases studies

Table		1	2	3	4	5	6
Type	Lockdown	No	No	Yes	Yes	Yes	Yes
	Vaccination	No	Yes	No	Yes	No	Yes
	Testing	High	High	Low	Low	High	High
Vaccination rate, v_k	Vulnerable nodes	0	0.02	0	0.02	0	0.02
	Robust nodes	0	0.01	0	0.01	0	0.01
Max testing capacity per day		20,000	20,000	5,000	5,000	20,000	20,000
Daily growth of testing = 3%, $\psi_T = 0.99$, $\psi_F = 0.22$, $\omega_{jk} \varepsilon (10^{-5}, 10^{-4})$, $W = 30$							

Population sizes and initial values for the nodes are in Table 5.3. The number of daily tests T_{kt} is assumed to grow daily by 3% until it reaches a maximum value.

We consider six scenarios described in Table 5.4. Comparative summaries, including across node maximums of peak hospitalization, deaths, and peak quarantined population, are displayed in Table 5.5. The optimal values of length, severity, and threshold parameters for imposing a lockdown, the resulting total economic cost, and total deaths, are displayed in Table 5.6.

Table 5.5 Maximum values of H, D, and Q among vulnerable and robust nodes, respectively. Percentages out of the population (for the node with the maximum value) are in parentheses

Scenario	Max H		Max D		Max Q	
	Vulnerable	Robust	Vulnerable	Robust	Vulnerable	Robust
1	55,258	7041	90,108	3684	56,151	31,029
	(12.28%)	(2.01%)	(20.02%)	(1.05%)	(12.48%)	(8.87%)
2	27,413	5327	49,494	2843	28,023	24,703
	(6.09%)	(1.52%)	(11.00%)	(0.81%)	(6.23%)	(7.06%)
3	604	1746	4210	2603	637	16,624
	(0.13%)	(0.05%)	(0.94%)	(0.74%)	(0.14%)	(4.75%)
4	1096	1749	2832	1836	893	13,163
	(0.24%)	(0.05%)	(0.63%)	(0.52%)	(0.02%)	(3.76%)
5	188	181	746 (0.17%)	194	198	1463
	(0.04%)	(0.05%)		(0.06%)	(0.04%)	(0.42%)
6	421	733	1061	664	461	5739
	(0.09%)	(0.21%)	(0.24%)	(0.19%)	(0.13%)	(1.64%)

Table 5.6 Optimal parameters and maximums of total lockdown duration for the vulnerable and robust are shown, respectively. The economic cost of lockdown (as annualized % of GDP) and total death of all nodes are also reported

Scenario	Optimal parameter		Max total lockdown duration (days)		Economic cost of lockdown (% of GDP)	Total death
	$(\kappa v, \kappa r)$	η	Vulnerable	Robust		
1	(1,1)	1	0	0	0	42,9137 (11.92%)
2	(1,1)	1	0	0	0	242,022 (6.72%)
3	(0.36, 0.36)	1×10^{-4}	387	368	57.32	30,272 (0.84%)
4	(0.25, 0.29)	3.57×10^{-4}	143	192	28.44	20,806 (0.58%)
5	(0.28, 7.76 × 10⁻⁵)	5.58×10^{-5}	317	305	63.25	3951 (0.11%)
6	(0.18, 0.23)	1.69×10^{-4}	115	152	24.73	7281 (0.20%)

A Shot at Herd Immunity

In the early days of the COVID-19 pandemic, a quick attainment of the herd immunity purely through recovery from infection without imposing any restrictions was considered to be a potentially "least economically disruptive" policy in many countries (e.g. Sweden, and at least initially the United Kingdom).

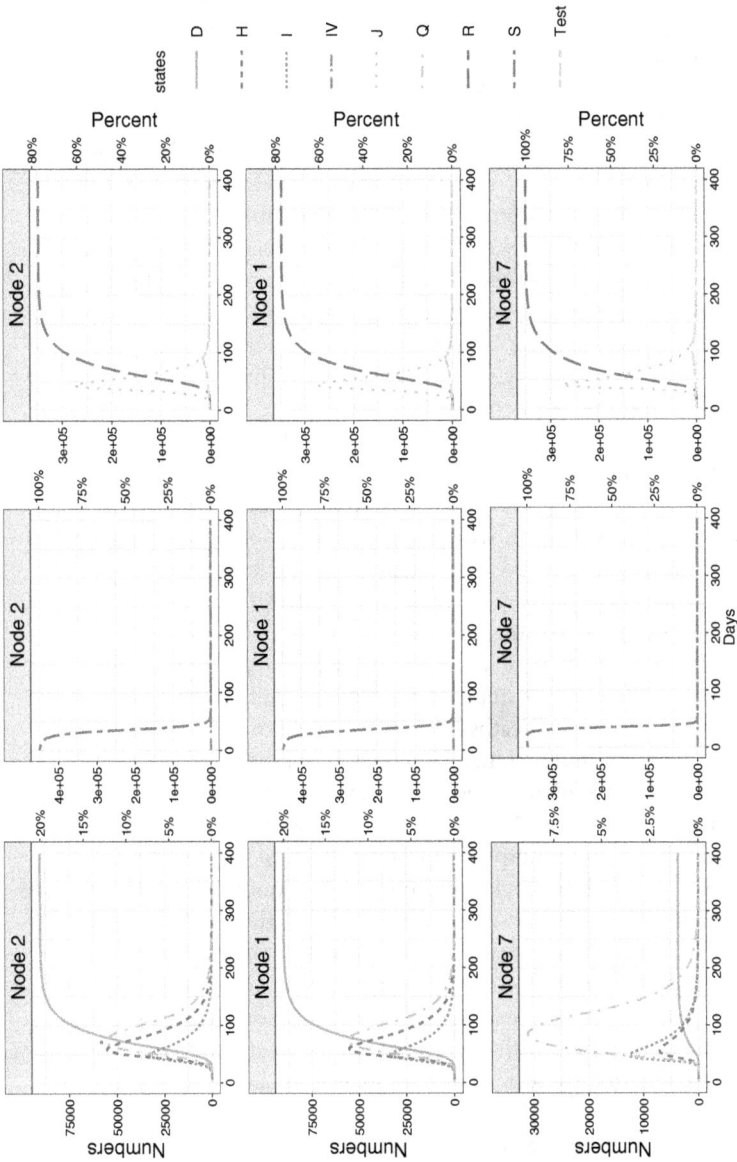

Figure 5.2 Scenario 1: Trajectories resulting from an attempt at achieving herd immunity with high level of testing, but without lockdown or vaccination

From Figures 5.2 and 5.3, the devastating cost of such a policy is evident. Without a lockdown, the number of susceptible falls exponentially fast, as essentially everyone in the population is exposed to the spread of the disease, and the pandemic runs its course within the first 100 days. This, however, comes at a terrible cost in terms of death and hospitalization. Without vaccination, even with high testing (Scenario 1), Tables 5.5 and 5.6, and Figure 5.2 show that approximately 12% of the population is likely to succumb to the disease. Death is particularly high amongst the vulnerable population, where nearly 20% of the people are expected to die. At its peak almost 12% and 2% of the population are expected to be hospitalized in the vulnerable and robust nodes, respectively. By any standards, these numbers paint a catastrophic picture and is well beyond the capacity of any country's healthcare system. The countries with large elderly and susceptible population are expected to be more severely hit. The Swedish policy of attaining a fast herd immunity has been controversial. It has severely stretched medical facilities, and it is largely accepted that Sweden has fared worse compared to other Scandinavian countries which chose a more conservative approach.

In addition, delayed introduction of a lockdown has resulted in severe shortage of hospital beds in countries including the United Kingdom (in 2020) and India (in 2021).

The introduction of vaccination on the 10th day after the onset (Scenario 2) does not improve the results significantly. Even though the total number of deaths has been reduced to 6.7%, it is still unacceptably high. In the vulnerable nodes, around 11% of the population perish. At the epidemic's peak, the hospitalization is about 6% in the vulnerable nodes and 1.5% in the robust nodes, which far exceeds the assumed maximum hospital capacity of 0.5% of the population.

Even though no lockdown means no economic cost due to loss of employment and business (see Table 5.6), the true cost of achieving a fast herd immunity is catastrophic. For simplicity, we exclude medical costs and closure of businesses due to infections (Ghosh, 2021, this volume). Assuming that each person dying has 30 additional years to live, with 11.92% death, the total cost to the economy is 357.6% and 201.6% of the annual GDP in Scenarios 1 and 2, respectively.

By comparing the economic costs of policies with optimal lockdown in Table 5.6, it becomes evident that the policy of achieving

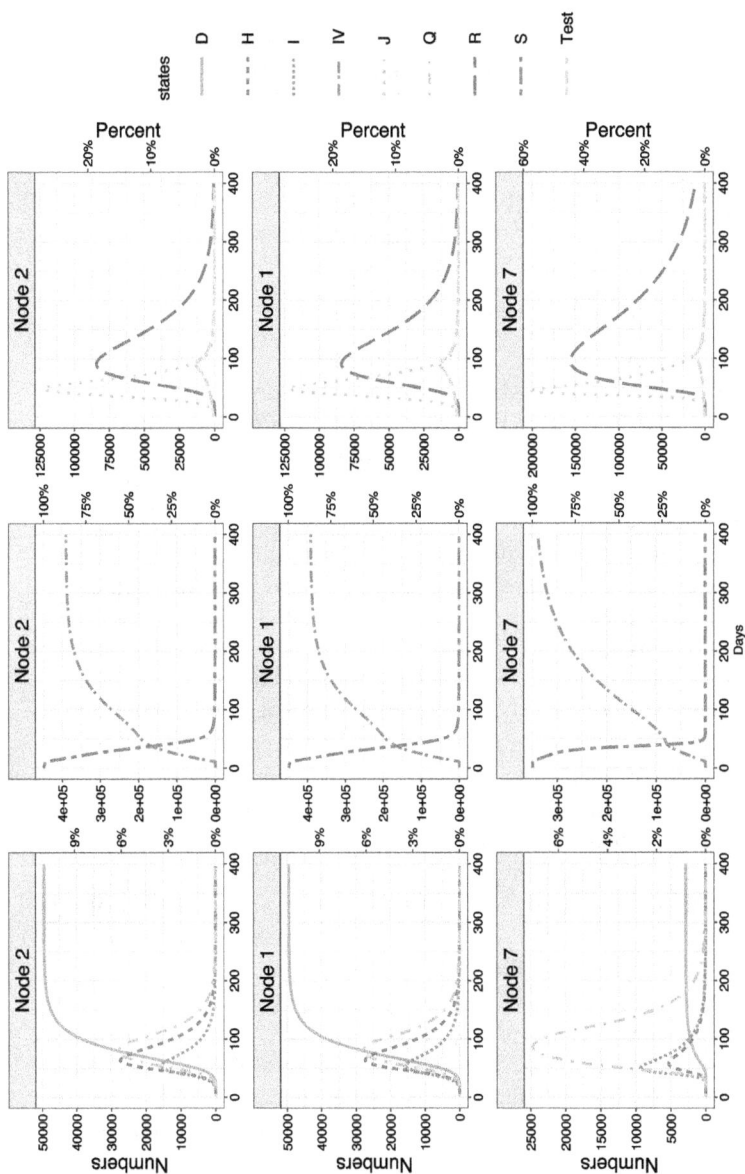

Figure 5.3 Scenario 2: Trajectories when no lockdown is allowed, but testing is high, and vaccination starts on the 10th day into the pandemic

herd immunity fast without a lockdown is not even economically viable.

In both Scenarios 1 and 2, the robust nodes are also severely affected. Comparing with the optimal values of (κ_v, κ_r) in other scenarios, it appears that a policy of isolating the vulnerable population with a lockdown, but leaving the robust population free of restrictions, does not seem to be viable either. Indeed, from the scenarios discussed below, it seems the optimal lockdown strategy is often harsher in the robust nodes than the vulnerable nodes.

Optimal Lockdown in a Low Testing Regime

The importance of mass testing and isolation of discovered cases through quarantines was emphasized by the WHO and several medical organizations from the early days of the pandemic. However, prevalence and effectiveness of testing in different countries have varied significantly. Countries like Taiwan, South Korea, Germany, and Iceland could scale up testing to cover a huge part of their population, while in many other countries, like the United Kingdom and India, a much smaller portion of the population could be tested.

In Scenarios 3 and 4, the daily testing was capped at 5,000 per node. Without the availability of vaccines, the proposed optimal strategy is to impose a long lockdown (387 days in vulnerable and 368 days in the robust nodes). The pandemic does not end within 400 days. But the susceptible population decreases quite slowly in the vulnerable nodes. In the robust nodes, the susceptible population initially decreases fast, followed by a sharp increase in latter stages, primarily due to migration (Figures 5.4 and 5.5).

The total mortality is low (0.84%); however, the peak hospitalization in the robust nodes reaches the maximum capacity of 0.5% (of the population). The peak quarantine rate is also quite high at 4.75%.

With vaccination starting on the 100th day, the situation shows a marked improvement. Short lockdown phases of 143 and 192 days, respectively, in the vulnerable and robust nodes, seem to reduce the number of susceptible persons fast, within 400 days. The lockdown

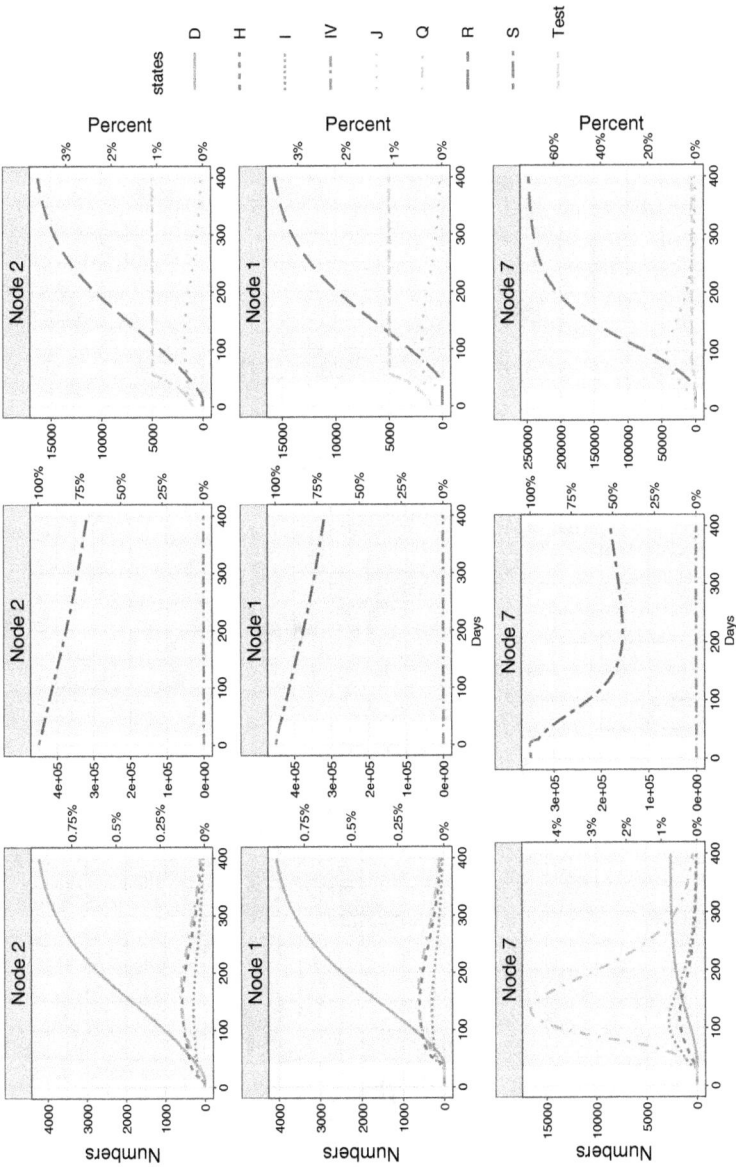

Figure 5.4 Scenario 3: Trajectories under a low testing regime and no vaccination

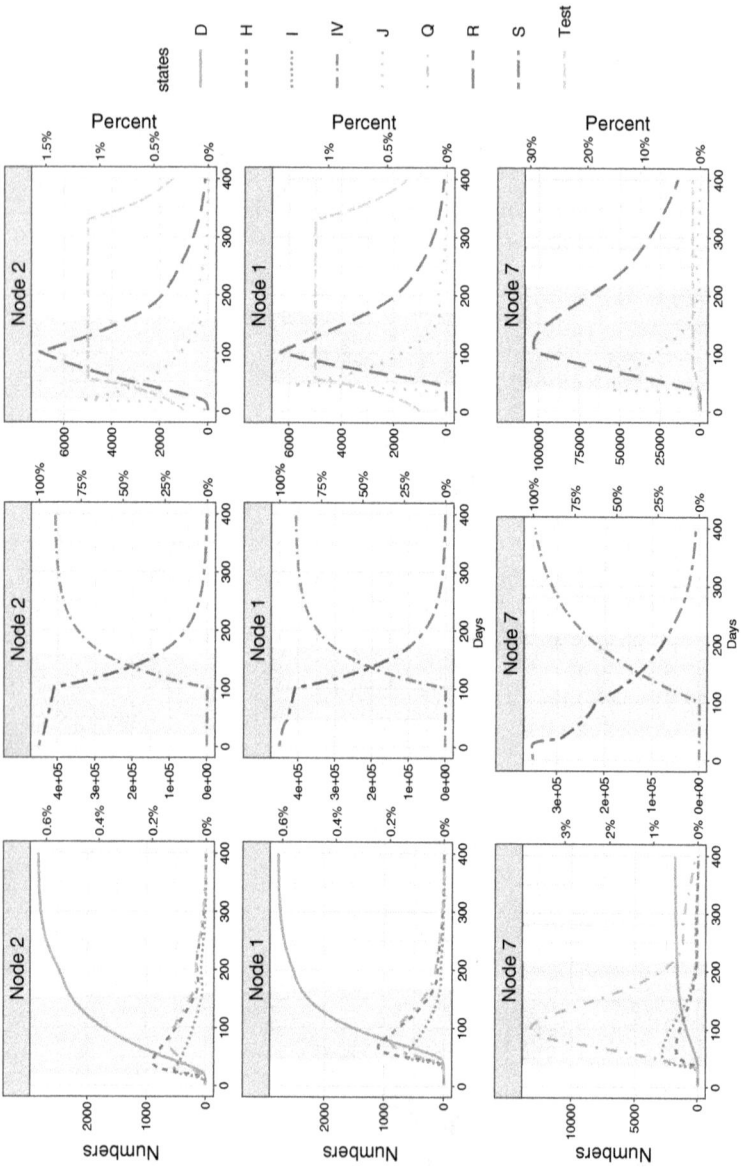

Figure 5.5 Scenario 4: Trajectories when vaccines are rolled out in a low testing regime

needs to be more severe than the settings with no vaccination (see Table 5.6). However, the economic cost due to lockdown is halved. The overall death percentage also reduces to 0.58%. Peak hospitalization in the robust nodes still reaches the assumed capacity (0.5%).

Optimal Lockdown in a High Testing Regime

We now consider the scenario where the maximum daily testing quickly increases daily by 3% to 20,000. With no vaccination, like in Scenarios 5, the pandemic does not end within 400 days. But, instead of a long, less severe lockdown, the optimal strategy involves repetitive lockdown phases, shown in Figure 5.6. The total lockdown duration is shorter than in Scenario 3, especially in the robust nodes. However, compared to Scenario 3, peak hospitalization rate and mortality are markedly lower. Even though fewer days are spent under lockdown, their increased severity (smaller (κ_v, κ_r)) results in a higher economic cost. Interestingly, the susceptible populations in the robust nodes actually show a slow increase.

With vaccination starting on the 100th day, the situation improves significantly. In Scenario 6, the optimal strategy involves a relatively modest initial lockdown period of 115 and 152 days in the vulnerable and robust nodes, respectively (Figure 5.7).

Once the vaccination starts, the susceptible population decreases exponentially, and the number of infected is reduced to zero within a year. Even though compared to Scenario 5, the number of deaths, peak hospitalizations, and peak quarantines are higher (see Table 5.5), the economic cost due to lockdown is much lower. In fact, it is even lower than the economic cost for Scenario 4.

DISCUSSION

Many aspects of the COVID-19 pandemic are still shrouded in mystery. The roll-out of several vaccines have provided some hope that the end of the pandemic might be near. This is especially true in the United States, where many restrictions, like mask wearing and social distancing, are being withdrawn.

Our case studies show that without mass vaccination, the pandemic will not end. However, this is not enough for controlling the

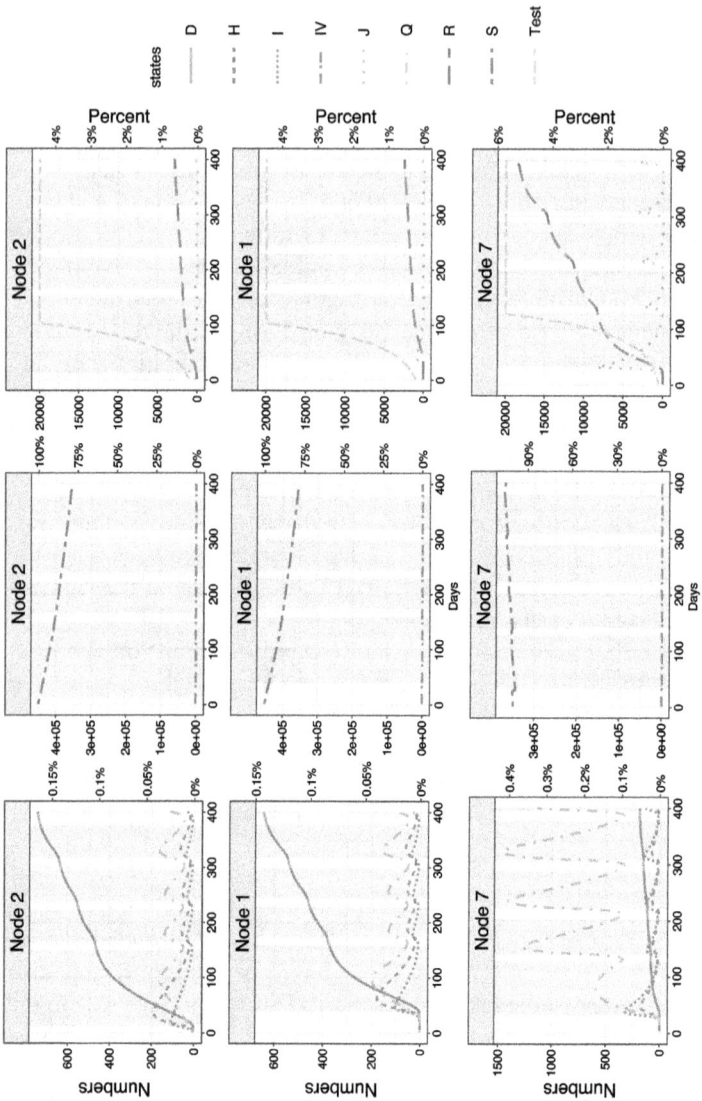

Figure 5.6 Scenario 5: Trajectories in a high testing paradigm, with no vaccination

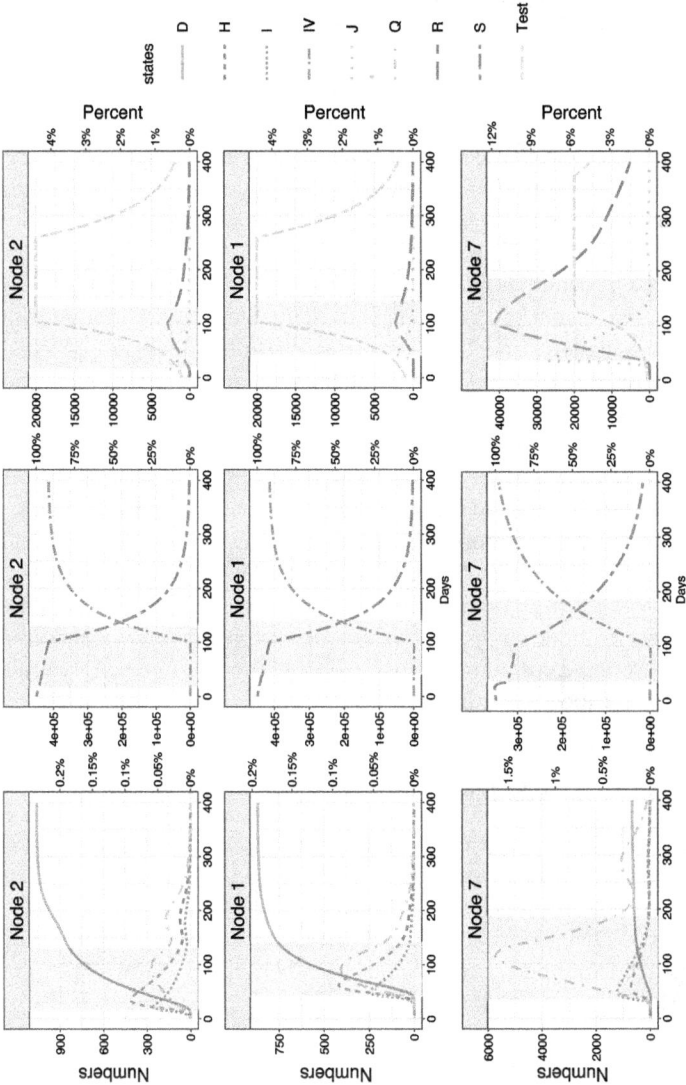

Figure 5.7 Scenario 6: Trajectories under a combination of high daily testing and vaccination

impact of the disease. Carefully designed lockdowns are very effective in dampening the spread of infections and providing relief to the healthcare system. Countries like Israel, the United Kingdom, Chile, and the United States have been able to achieve a high vaccination rate. However, given the uncertainty in the effectiveness of the vaccines in preventing infections by mutant forms of the virus, the necessity of imposing periodic lockdown remains.

Our study clearly demonstrates the disastrous consequences of the strategy of attaining "herd immunity". In fact, except for Sweden, no country seems to have chosen that path. The positive effects of a strict lockdown in controlling the pandemic in a relatively short time were observed in countries like China, Australia, and New Zealand. Similarly, many countries like Spain, Iran, Italy, Denmark, Germany, the United Kingdom, and India have imposed multiple phases of lockdown, not as a containment strategy, but to address immediate healthcare crises.

Our analyses show that a combination of "mundane" strategies like extensive diagnostic testing, periodic lockdown, and vaccination is the key to control and finally eradicate a destabilizing pandemic like COVID-19. Furthermore, optimal strategies can be devised to minimize the economic cost due to lockdown, limit the number of deaths, and relieve the stress on the health infrastructure. By modifying migration policies, node compositions, and the relative importance of deaths in the proposed cost function, the proposed model can be used to suit many population structures and scenarios that may emerge in future.

ACKNOWLEDGEMENTS

The authors would like to thank Professor Prabir Burman for helpful discussions. Grant support: Shuting Liao (NASA-TRISH 19-19BRASH-2-0055); Debashis Paul (NSF DMS-1713120, DMS-1811405, DMS-1915894, NASA-TRISH 19-19BRASH-2-0055); Sanjay Chaudhuri (MoE Singapore R155000194114, R15500 0215114). Joint first author: S.B., S.L.; Contribution: S.B., S.L. Coding, Simulation, Manuscript Preparation; D.P., S.C. Formulation, Editing; S.B. S.C. Algorithm.

NOTE

This contributed chapter was accepted for publication in this refereed edited volume on July 1, 2021.

REFERENCES

Badr, H. S., et al., (2020), "Association between mobility patterns and COVID-19 transmission in the USA: a mathematical modelling study," *The Lancet Infectious Diseases*, 20(11), pp. 1247–1254.

Bhattacharjee, S., et al., (2021), "Inference on the dynamics of the covid pandemic from observational data," medRxiv.

Brett, T. S. and P. Rohani, (2020), "Transmission dynamics reveal the impracticality of COVID-19 herd immunity strategies," *Proceedings of the National Academy of Sciences*, 117(41), pp. 25897–25903.

Bubar, K. M., et al., (2021), "Model-informed COVID-19 vaccine prioritization strategies by age and serostatus," *Science*, 371(6532), pp. 916–921.

Cirakli, U., et al., (2021), "The relationship between COVID-19 cases and COVID-19 testing: a panel data analysis on OECD countries," *Journal of the Knowledge Economy*, pp. 1–14.

Giordano, G., et al., (2020), "Modelling the COVID-19 epidemic and implementation of population-wide interventions in Italy," *Nature medicine*, 26(6), pp. 855–860.

Ghosh, A., (2022), "Is Life vs Livelihood a False Choice?"," In *Managing Complexity and Covid-19: Life, Liberty Or The Pursuit of Happiness*, Edited by A. Ghosh, A. Haldar and K. Bhaumik, Routledge, pp. 3–19.

Ivorra, B., et al., (2020), "Mathematical modelling of the spread of the coronavirus disease 2019 (COVID-19) taking into account the undetected infections. The case of China," *Communications in Nonlinear Science and Numerical Simulation*, 88, 105303.

Kucharski, A. J., et al., (2020), "Early dynamics of transmission and control of COVID-19: a mathematical modelling study," *The lancet infectious diseases*, 20(5), pp. 553–558.

Kwok, K. O., et al., (2020), "Herd immunity – estimating the level required to halt the COVID-19 epidemics in affected countries," *Journal of Infection*, 80(6), e32–e33.

Mbwogge, M., (2021), "Mass testing with contact tracing compared to test and trace for the effective suppression of COVID-19 in the United Kingdom: systematic review," *JMIRx Med*, 2(2), e27254.

Prem, K., et al., (2020), "The effect of control strategies to reduce social mixing on outcomes of the COVID-19 epidemic in Wuhan, China: a modelling study," *The Lancet Public Health*, 5(5), e261–e270.

Randolph, H. E. and L. B. Barreiro, (2020), "Herd immunity: understanding COVID-19," *Immunity*, 52(5), pp. 737–741.

Soltesz, K., et al., (2020), "The effect of interventions on COVID-19," *Nature*, 588(7839), E26–E28.

Susskind, D. and D. Vines, (2020), "The economics of the COVID-19 pandemic: an assessment," *Oxford Review of Economic Policy*, 36(Supplement_1), S1–S13.

Tolles, J. and T. Luong, (2020), "Modelling epidemics with compartmental models," *JAMA*, 323(24), pp. 2515–2516.

6

VIRTUAL FIRESIDE CONVERSATIONS WITH BUSINESS LEADERS

With Co-Editors Aurobindo Ghosh (AG), Amit Haldar (AH), and Kalyan Bhaumik (KB)

Conversation with **Sourav Ganguly (SG), President of Board of Control for Cricket in India and Former Captain, Indian Cricket Team**

Cricket historian Boria Majumdar mused about global icons from West Bengal in India, "There are three Bengalis who are global brands who will stand the test of time—[Nobel Laureate poet] Rabindranath Tagore, [Lifetime Oscar winning director] Satyajit Ray and Sourav Ganguly." The latter being the second most winningest former India cricket captain and current Board of Control for Cricket in India (BCCI) President (Sardesai, 2017, p. 250). Being the only living icon of the trio entails a tremendous responsibility, and of course expectations, not just in West Bengal but also in India and the cricketing world. Cricket is not just the second most popular game in the world after football, with more than 2.5 billion people playing and watching it (Shvili, 2020), but it is like a religion in the Indian subcontinent. The Indian Premier League (IPL), the fourth most profitable but the fastest growing sports league in the world, that showcases young cricketing talent in India and abroad hosted by the BCCI, a multi-billion-dollar statutory board, was hit by COVID-19 like every other industry (Randjelovic, 2020). In the thick of a devastating pandemic, BCCI President Ganguly and his leadership team contemplated and successfully hosted the 2020 edition of the

DOI: 10.4324/9781003218807-7

IPL in the UAE in an unprecedented bio-bubble with stringent COVID-safe protocol being adhered to. However, with cases going down in February 2021, there was renewed hope it can be hosted at home in the cricket-mad country of origin with limited or no spectators, when the unexpected "tsunami of infections" in the second wave hit. Despite bravely trying, the tournament had to be halted after a breach of the bio-bubble with multiple players coming down with the disease. The editors of Managing Complexity and COVID-19 virtually interviewed BCCI President Sourav Ganguly, for whom another English cricketing stalwart, Geoff Boycott, have given the epithet of "the Prince of Kolkata," to hear his views on the impact of the pandemic on sports, on the aspirations of young athletes in the country where the main live entertainment outlet is to watch cricket.

1. How can one look after the financial health of a sports organization in such troubled times? What about the other organizations of the country? Any suggestions for them?

SG: It depends on the sports organization, to be honest. Some organizations are very sound like the cricket board (BCCI) for which COVID-19 has not affected the finances significantly at all. Some of the most successful leagues around the world have remained the same despite the pandemic. So, the financial well-being of the organization depends on how strong the foundation of that sports is in the country. It also depends on the individual's financial management style, so I don't think there is any hard and fast rule.

2. What's your idea about a spectator-less match? How does it affect the fans and the players? If it's only for TV, is a single venue preferable to multiple venues?

SG: I think it's not the best thing for anybody to have a spectator-less match. Players want to see the spectators; players want to see stands full and players want to hear the applause for a good shot or a famous victory. It also affects the fans who want to see live cricket, but they are not allowed entry, due to the strict restrictions. So, it is not an easy thing for them, at all. For the players, as I said, it's difficult for them to play in front of empty stands but for TV audience, it doesn't matter. TV brings the game right into your bedrooms, and drawing rooms, so it doesn't affect viewership for television.

3. How are young players affected because of this pandemic? Do you have any advice for them?

SG: Young players are, of course, affected by this pandemic. They are not able to play the sport that they love and for such a long time; it becomes quite unbearable. It has been for almost 15 months that these young players have not been able to play the game. The restrictions have protected them against the virus that can affect their physical health and lives. Unfortunately, that's the way it has been for the entire time, I feel, it has taken a toll on them mentally.

4. What are the factors that you kept in mind while organizing tournaments, in the midst of the pandemic? What factors did you keep in mind while choosing the venues on both occasions?

SG: The most important thing that you want to take care of during the pandemic is health and safety. The bio-bubbles are made and kept under strict protocols. The players and organizers are kept away from contacting other people and outsiders. So, it creates a "known zone" where not many people are in contact with them because nobody knows who is carrying the virus. Hence, creating bio-bubbles and creating a safety zone are very important for the smooth running of the league and tournament.

5. Why is maintaining a biosafety bubble so difficult?

SG: Maintaining a bio-bubble is obviously difficult because it requires a lot of discipline. It requires staying in a room day in and day out. It affects people mentally to stay in a completely enclosed environment, not to see your own friends. The players cannot go out to get fresh air. We often take it for granted, but not having that independence is really quite daunting. So, from that point of view, maintaining a safety bio-bubble is not an easy thing.

6. What are the lessons learnt from these experiences that can be useful for future sports organizers?

SG: Well, you know this is a pandemic, you learn a lot of lessons. Most importantly, you just say to yourself and pray to the Almighty and hope that it doesn't come back again. If this pandemic continues year after year, it's a massive threat to human society. For all of us, we all pray and hope that it's done and dusted.

7. What will be the long-lasting effects of this pandemic on sports?

SG: We are in the middle of the second wave and that also is going down in terms of numbers all around the country and most importantly, around the world. We need to get back to normalcy, that's what we live for and that's what we all want. I don't think any of us expect this disruption to occur again.

NOTE

This contributed chapter was accepted for publication in this refereed edited volume on June 21, 2021.

REFERENCES

Randjelovic, D., (2020), "11 MOST PROFITABLE SPORTS LEAGUES – THEIR VALUE WILL SURPRISE YOU," https://apsportseditors.org/others/most-profitable-sports-leagues/.

Sardesai, R., (2017), *Democracy's XI: The Great Indian Cricket Story*, Juggernaut Books, India.

Shvili, J., (2020), "The Most Popular Sports in the World," The World Atlas, https://www.worldatlas.com/articles/what-are-the-most-popular-sports-in-the-world.html.

PART II

THERAPY UNDER UNCERTAINTY

Medical Perspective in a Pandemic

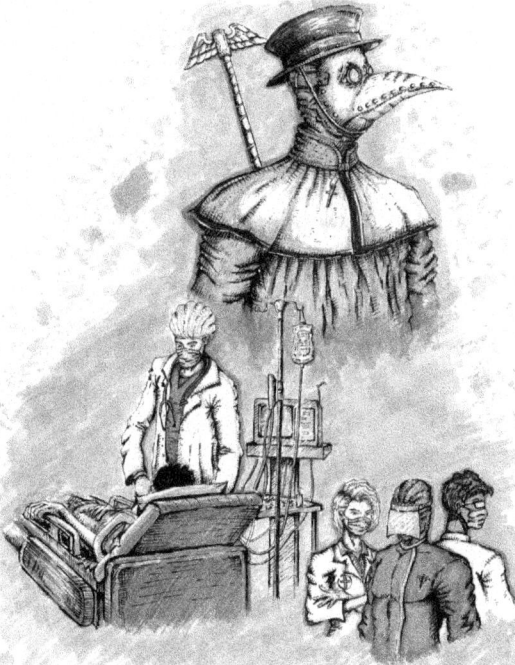

7

NAVIGATING AN UNCHARTERED SEA

Finding the Right Test and Testing Pathway

Amit Haldar

...Sit down before a fact as a little child, ...follow humbly wherever and to whatever abysses nature leads, or you shall learn nothing...

Thomas Huxley (Barry, 2005)

INTRODUCTION

In the winter of 2019, Dr Li Wenliang, an ophthalmologist working at Wuhan Central Hospital in China was the first person to warn his colleagues about a suspected outbreak of an illness that resembled severe acute respiratory syndrome (SARS). The clinical characteristics of these patients bore resemblance to those observed during the outbreak of SARS-CoV-1, which emerged in 2002–2003 and had caused more than 8,000 confirmed cases and approximately 800 deaths. The authorities initially refused to acknowledge the outbreak (Green, 2020). Soon, this episode of SARS spread like wildfire across the globe resulting in a pandemic of devastating proportions.

On 31 December 2019, the Chinese CDC (Centre for Disease Control) despatched a rapid response team to conduct an epidemiologic and aetiological (causative) investigation along with the local authorities. They collected lower respiratory tract samples including bronchoalveolar lavage fluid from some of the affected persons. The scientists extracted nuclei acid from the clinical samples and subjected

DOI: 10.4324/9781003218807-9

the samples to advanced techniques of molecular biology including **polymerase chain reaction (PCR)**. The causative agent was soon found to be a spherical enveloped single-stranded RNA virus belonging to the Coronaviradae family. The similarities of the isolated virus to the one that caused the SARS outbreak (SARSCoVs) led the Coronavirus Study Group of the International Committee on Taxonomy of Viruses to term the virus as SARS-CoV-2 (Cascella et al., 2020). The associated disease was named as COVID-19 (Acronym for Corona Virus Disease, 19, recognizes the year of recognition).

THE SARS-COV2 VIRUS

The virion (singular of virus) has four principal structural proteins that are essential for assembly of the virion and its associated infective capacity (Mousavizadeh et al., 2021). These are S (Spike), E (Envelope), M (Membrane), and N (Nucleocapsid) (Figure 7.1).

Homotrimers (a protein that consists of three identical polypeptide units) of S proteins make up the spikes on the viral surface. These are responsible for attachment to receptors on the host cells. The S protein consists of two subunits, S1 and S2. These are separately responsible for the viral attachment and membrane fusion

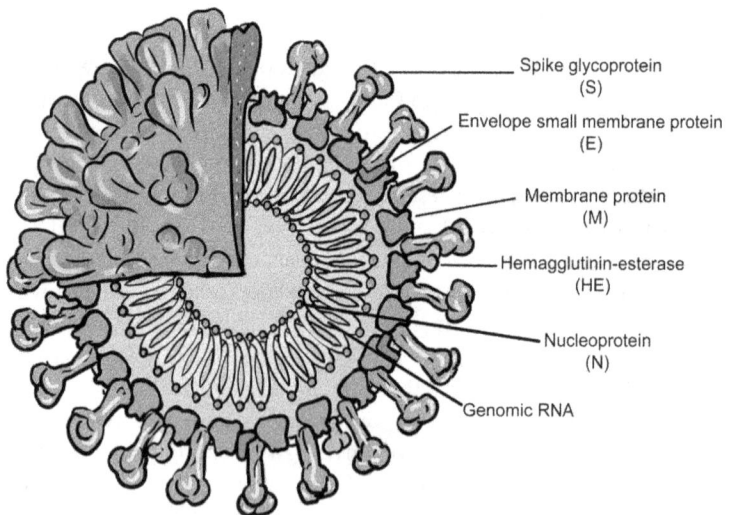

Figure 7.1 SARS COV2, schematic

during entry of the virus into its host cell. The main host receptor involved in the process of attachment of the spike protein is the ACE2 (Hoffmann et al., 2020). The M protein has three transmembrane domains and shapes the virion, promotes membrane curvature, and covers the nucleocapsid. The E protein participates in virus assembly and release, and is involved in viral pathogenesis. The N protein presents two domains, both of which can bind virus RNA genome via different mechanisms. There are certain accessory proteins like HE protein, 3A/B protein, and 4A/B protein.

Respiratory viruses usually infect either the throat or the lungs. Those that concentrate in the throat cause milder symptoms but spread very easily. Viruses that penetrate the lungs cause more severe illness but are much less infectious. SARS-CoV-2 is both very contagious and at the same time aggressive. There is something unique about the SARS-Cov2 genetic sequence that renders it highly infectious and capable of involving multiple targets This is a **unique nucleotide sequence (ccu cgg cgg gca)** in its genome. The virus's 12 extra letters create a site in the spike protein that can be cleaved by the **furin** enzyme which is present in almost all human cells. This can explain why the virus is so highly virulent and contagious. The manner in which the SARS-COV2 virus acquired this extra nucleotide sequence (when jumping species) is yet to be known and remains a subject of speculation (Ansede, 2020).

TESTING

Isolation of the organism by culture of a specimen obtained from the infected host is the traditional method as described in Koch,s (Robert Koch, the German physician and father of microbiology) postulate. But viral cultures are cumbersome and expensive. Molecular biology has advanced and can allow detection of one or more of the proteins present in the body of the organism (Antigen test). The method used most frequently during the present pandemic of COVID-19 has been the direct detection of nucleic acids or detection via amplification of nuclei acids (NAAT) (Fredericks and Relman, 1996). Amongst the NAATs, **RT-PCR** (Reverse Transcriptase-Polymerase Chain Reaction) has emerged as the gold standard in diagnosis of COVID-19.

Apart from these direct tests, there are indirect tests that study the effects of these pathogens on the body. These are known as serological or immunological tests. They depend on the presence of antibodies in the blood. These antibodies appear as a response of the body against the invading foreign pathogen. Once the antibodies appear, the active phase of the infection usually ends. The antibodies commonly tested are the immunoglobulins. IgM usually appear first, followed by the IgG. These antibodies are usually directed against the different viral antigens or proteins (capsular or spike). Different antibodies may therefore have different protective ability. In fact, the S protein is the main inducer of a neutralizing antibody. There are also other markers of the cell-mediated immune response.

DIRECT TESTS

Direct tests involve obtaining samples from the appropriate tissues and then subjecting these specimens to culture or tests of molecular biology.

A variety of RNA gene targets have been used by different manufacturers in case of SARS-Cov2 for amplification, with most tests targeting 1 or more of the envelopes (*env*), nucleocapsid (*N*), spike (*S*), RNA-dependent RNA *polymerase (RdRp)*, and *ORF1* genes (Corman et al., 2020).

RT-PCR

The sample obtained person's nasopharynx or oropharynx is transported in the **liquid viral transport media (**Hanks' balanced salt, 0.4% fetal bovine serum, HEPES, antibiotic and antifungal agents) to the lab. The RNA is extracted and then reverse-transcribed to DNA (reverse because DNA to RNA conversion is termed "transcription" in biochemical parlance) by an enzyme called reverse transcriptase. This is because DNA can be copied. After that complementary DNA fragments are added to specific parts of the transcribed DNA. If the virus is present in this sample, the complementary fragments attach themselves to target sections of viral DNA.

The mixture is then placed in the RT-PCR machine with the addition of reagents and subjected to temperature-controlled process of denaturing (double-stranded template DNA is heated to separate into two fragments), annealing (cooling allows DNA primers to attach to template DNA), and extending (new strand of DNA made). The whole process is termed as a cycle. This cycle is repeated 35 to 45 times to continue copying of sections of viral DNA creating around 35 billion copies of the target DNA. Marker labels attach to the DNA strands and release a fluorescent dye, which is measured by the computer and presented in real time on the screen (Figure 7.2).

The number of cycles of the amplification reaction needed for the confirmation of the presence of virus is termed as **cycle threshold (Ct)**. Higher the viral load, lower is the Ct value to confirm positivity. This Ct value is dependent on a number of variables. They include the assay's gene target, the extraction platform, PCR amplification chemistry, and even the quality of specimen collection. The inherent sensitivity of real-time PCR allows for detection of minute amounts (e.g., <100 copies/ml) of target nucleic acid in clinical samples (Binnicker et al., 2020).

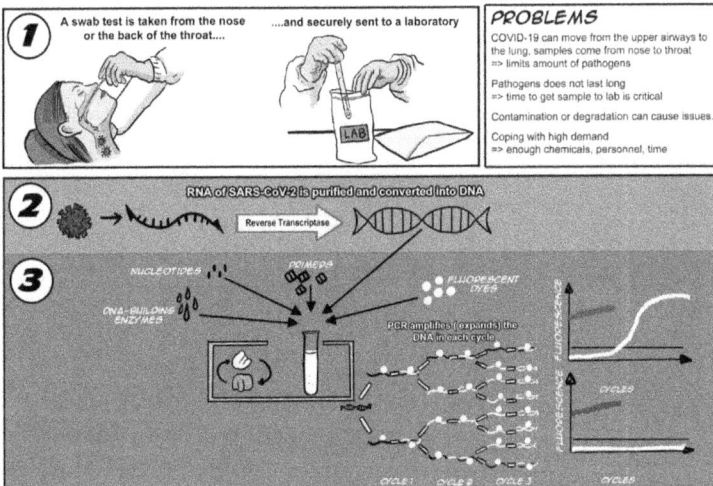

Figure 7.2 Steps in polymerase chain reaction

OBTAINING THE RIGHT SAMPLE

The virus seems to have a high affinity for the cells of the respiratory tract. Nasopharyngeal swabs (60–70% sensitivity) and upper airway specimens are the most commonly used sample. However, sputum (73% sensitivity) or bronchoalveolar lavage fluid (93%) (a specimen from the lower airway/ lungs) obtained by bronchoscopy may have higher sensitivity according to some studies. A later, small hospital cohort study among patients with laboratory-confirmed COVID-19 reported that the positivity rate of RT-PCR for SARS-CoV-2 is 15–30% in blood and 14–38% in rectal swabs (Wang et al., 2020).

TIMING IS THE KEY

The viral RNA obtained from the nasopharyngeal swab is detectable by the PCR as early as day 1 of symptoms and peaks within the first week of symptom onset. A specimen obtained from the nasopharynx around day 5 after the symptom onset has the maximum sensitivity. The positivity starts to decline by the 3rd week and then becomes negative. In a minority of patients, however, viral fragments can remain detectable for up to 2 months and beyond after the initial infection. Positivity in such cases does not signify infectivity (Figure 7.3).

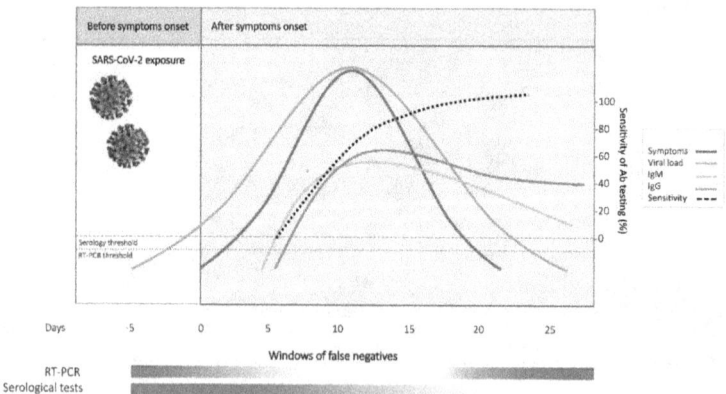

Figure 7.3 Timing of the viral tests

TECHNIQUE

Right collection technique is of utmost importance and should be performed by a trained laboratory person wearing adequate PPE (personal protection equipment).

LIMITATIONS

The RT-PCR method involves technical expertise, skilled lab technicians, and a PCR machine. False negatives can occur due to wrong timing of collection, poor quality of specimen, inappropriate handling and shipment, and technical errors in running the test. It is time consuming and may take up to 6 hours to complete the stipulated 45 cycles. If the PCR technique is done in an automated fashion, the turnaround time (TAT) may be reduced by half.

MODIFICATIONS

Gen X pert assay (CB-NAAT) is a modification of the conventional RT-PCR where the test is done in a cartridge based (CB) system with pre-added reagents needed for the amplification reaction. There is no need for prior RNA extraction in this method. Hence, the results can be obtained in an hour. It is more expensive.

In India, True Nat, a portable version of CB Nat, has been approved by the Indian Council of Medical Research (ICMR) for use. The advantage of True Nat is that the machines used for the test are smaller, portable, and battery operated. This allows teams to set up mobile testing centres or kiosks in containment zones, instead of having to transport samples to labs. Earlier, True NAT has been used in India for diagnosis of tuberculosis (Basu, 2020).

POOLING OF SAMPLES

Testing of sample pools (combining respiratory samples from several people and conducting one test) has been suggested as a solution to increase the testing of samples, while maintaining test sensitivity and specificity. This can be done in two ways:

1   Sample/media pooling: Pooling aliquots of transport media each containing a single patient sample

or

2   Swab pooling: Adding swabs from multiple patients into a single volume of transport media

If the pooled sample tests negative, all the tested individuals are considered negative for COVID-19. If the pooled test is positive, then all the individual samples in the pool need to be tested.

This is specifically useful in settings where the incidence of infection is low. It has been used in screening workers returning to work or students coming back to school after a gap (CDC, 2020).

NEWER TECHNOLOGIES

Point-of-care (POC) tests are being developed to offset the disadvantages of RT-PCR.

They include an in vitro automated assay that utilizes isothermal nucleic acid amplification technology for the qualitative detection of SARS-CoV-2 viral nucleic acids. They can provide results within 13 minutes.

A team of scientists in India developed an inexpensive paper-based test for coronavirus that could provide fast results similar to a pregnancy test. The test, named after a famous Indian fictional detective (**FELUDA** = Acronym for FnCas9 Editor Linked Uniform Detection Assay)), is based on a gene-editing technology called **CRISPR**. (Acronym for Clustered Regularly Interspaced Short Palindromic Repeats). RAY (short for Rapid variant AssaY), a faster variant of FELUDA, has been developed but has not gained popularity due its slightly higher cost (Biswas et al., 2020).

It is somewhat similar to SHERLOCK (Specific high sensitivity enzymatic reporter unlocking) which has been developed by scientists from the Broad Institute in the United States. However, FELUDA does not need a reporter and is less complex.

ANTIGEN TESTS

Antigen tests detect viral antigens or proteins. These can be done rapidly and are inexpensive POC tests. Most rapid antigen tests

(RAT or ART) are primarily fluorescent immunoassays. The antigenic target is the nucleocapsid protein (as it is the most abundant viral protein). The same nasopharyngeal swab is used in majority.

METHODOLOGY FOR THE ANTIGEN TESTS

There is usually a kit whose contents are the test device, specimen extraction buffer tube, sterile swab for sample collection, and nozzle cap. The nasopharyngeal swab sample is collected and placed in the buffer tube. Drops of the extracted specimen is then placed in the specimen well of the prepared test device. After 15 to 20 minutes, the test device is inserted into the analyzer which automatically scans and displays the results.

Results can be obtained in 30 minutes. The sensitivity of these tests is variable and less in comparison to the amplification tests like RT-PCR. Therein comes the question what level of sensitivity and specificity is acceptable for the RATs?

According to the ICMR guidelines issued on 19.05.21, minimum acceptance criteria of sensitivity and specificity of rapid Ag test kits include:

- Validated as a point-of-care test (POCT) without transport to a laboratory setup:
  Sensitivity: 50% and above; Specificity: 95% and above
- Validated in a laboratory setup with samples collected in viral transport medium (VTM):
  Sensitivity: 70% and above; Specificity: 99% and above

Self-testing may be possible with some of the kits. As the sensitivity of the antigen tests continue to improve, this can be of use in rapidly identifying and isolating persons attending functions or other group activities (e.g. sports).

The main purpose is to test and isolate the possible infected individual and prevent potential spread at an early stage while waiting for the confirmatory PCR test results. This testing protocol helps to control secondary spread better by accelerating contact tracing and is being used extensively in some countries like Singapore (Chong, 2021).

INDIRECT TESTS

Indirect tests are the tests that detect antibodies. They start becoming positive when the body immune response starts acting. The median seroconversion rates of total antibodies, IgM, and IgG were 11, 12, and 14 days. The cumulative seroconversion curve suggests that the rate for total antibody and IgM reached 100% within 30 days after the onset of ELISA-based IgM and IgG antibody tests have greater than 95% specificity for diagnosis of COVID-19. The antibody is detected from blood (Zhao et al., 2020).

So, these serological tests may be more useful in detecting past infection. This can also give us an idea about how long the immunity will stay after a given infection. Response to a particular vaccine can also be assessed by measuring the antibody levels. However, absence of antibodies after vaccination does not signify failure of the immune response and vice versa.

ROLE OF RADIOLOGY

Amongst the indirect tests, the radiological tests have played an important role not only in diagnosis but also in understanding the severity of disease. Computerized tomography (CT) scan of the chest can be a useful screening tool for diagnosis of viral pneumonia in the early stage of the disease. Recent studies have shown that the CT imaging can demonstrate typical characteristic radiological findings such as multiple ground-glass opacities, patchy pulmonary consolidations, and crazy-paving pattern, typically involving peripheral, sub-pleural, and basal areas of the lungs (Figure 7.4).

A retrospective study found the detection rate of baseline chest CT was more sensitive (98%) than baseline RT-PCR (71%). The overall sensitivity, specificity, NPV (negative predictive value), and diagnostic accuracy of the initial CT scan were 100%, 28%, 100%, and 71%, respectively (Bollineni et al., 2021).

LIMITATIONS

The radiological finings of COVID-19 pneumonia may overlap with other viral pneumonia. Hence, the positive predictive value depends on the stage of the epidemic and prevalence of other

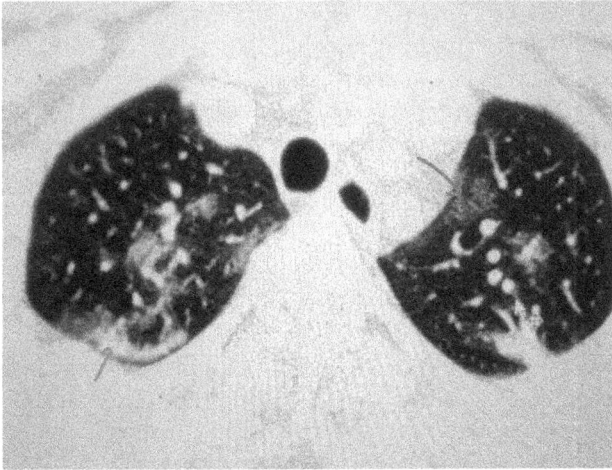

Figure 7.4 The COVID lungs with GGO and consolidation

pneumonias. The reading is also dependent on the expertise of the radiologist. CT scan of the chest is an expensive test and may not be available in a remote facility.

CT scan causes exposure of body to the radiation. Modern chest CT scans deliver about 6–7 milliSv (Sievert is a derived unit of ionizing radiation dose in the International System of Units). This is 60 to 70 times more than a chest X-ray. The lifetime risk of developing cancer after one CT scan of the chest is less than 1 in 3,000.

Newer screening techniques may reduce the radiation dose of CT scans even further.

TESTING PROTOCOL

Rapid Antigen Tests (RATs) and RT-PCR tests are therefore more useful before the onset of symptoms (pre-symptomatic) or at the early symptomatic stage in identifying the disease. The role of CT scans also needs to be overemphasized in this stage of the disease. However, while the efficacy of the nasopharyngeal swab test gradually drops off around 2–3 weeks after the onset of symptoms, serology-based tests are only feasible once antibodies appear in the blood. They can be detected in the serum 1–2 weeks after then onset of symptoms.

In a study by Guo et al., during the first 5.5 days, quantitative PCR had a higher positivity rate than IgM, whereas IgM ELISA had a higher positivity rate after day 5.5 of illness (Guo et al., 2020).

Given the sensitivity (correctly detecting a positive COVID-19 infection) and the specificity (correctly rejecting a false COVID-19 infection) of the various test results, the RT-PCR and serology tests often complement each other (Seethuraman et al., 2020).

The role of the antibody testing is going to become more and more important as vaccination continues. Those who have high antibody titers are less likely to be infected. If infected, they usually have a much more mild disease (See, 2021).

Community serological surveillance thus may be useful in assessing progress towards herd immunity and thus chalk out the road map for vaccination. It can also give us an idea about how long the immunity can last after vaccination (Ghosh et al., 2022).

One additional complication is the significant possibility of transmission from asymptomatic or more likely pre-symptomatic carriers (Statnews, 2020). For example, just to manage the risk of unwitting spread of COVID-19 with possibly more infectious variants in Phase II heightened alert stage, countries like Singapore have instituted new rules. These rules isolate patients whose RAT comes out to be positive while the patients are waiting for the PCR test results.

The suitability of a particular test depends on its sensitivity, specificity, timing, cost, and availability.

A few illustrative examples will help us to understand when to test, whom to test, and what to test.

CASE 1

A 55-year-old male is brought to the emergency with 3-day history of fever and breathlessness. His oxygen saturation is 94% in room air. His pulse rate is 100/min, BP130/80.

Q1) Does the patient need admission?

Q2) What tests to do?

Ans1) Considering the short history, this patient needs admission as the patient is symptomatic and his oxygen saturation is tending to decrease. But his admission can be done in the ward for observation till the full investigation reports come.

Ans 2) The emergency physician has to keep COVID-19 amongst the list of his differential diagnosis.

On D3 of the disease, RT-PCR may or may not be positive. It should be sent, but the report may be delayed by 12 hours. If a CB-NAAT is available, it should be sent as the results are available in an hour. But, if it is not available, a RAT may be done.

Routine blood tests like complete blood count, CRP (and markers of inflammation like IL6 and Serum Ferritin), and D-dimer (screening for coagulopathy) should be tested. Routine blood biochemistry including sugar, urea, creatinine, liver function tests, and urine routine examination may be done.

Q3) What happens if the CB—NAAT or RAT comes negative?

If RAT is negative, one should wait for NAAT. But if NAAT is also negative, a CT chest may be done. If CT is not available, chest radiography can provide clues. The sensitivity of chest radiography increases over time in the case of COVID-19 from 55% at Day ≤ 2 to 79% at Day > 11 after symptom onset (Stephanie et al., 2020). Treatment should be continued till the tests (including RT-PCR) are repeated after 3 to 4 days.

Q4) What will happen to the patient in a rural healthcare set-up?

Getting a NAAT done in a rural set-up is difficult. If RAT is not available, then the physician has to rely on his clinical judgement to come to a diagnosis. Apart from the routine blood tests, chest X-ray may be the only tool available in a resource-poor setting.

CASE 2

A 40-year-old laboratory worker was afflicted by SARI (severe acute respiratory illness). His RT-PCR was done from a nasopharyngeal swab on Day-5 of the illness. It came back negative for SARS-Cov2. He continued to worsen and was hospitalized as his oxygen saturation levels dropped to 88% in room air. CT scan showed evidence of moderate lung involvement. He was started on systemic steroids and antibiotics.

Q1) What to do next?

A repeat RT-PCR sample needs to be sent after 2–3 days.

In a retrospective study of 610 hospitalized patients from Wuhan, Li et al. found that of the 39.5% were confirmed to be tested for COVID-19 by the RT-PCR. However, only 27.5% came back positive on the first test. 0.2% were weakly positive, and 9.3% were dubious positive. Second, third, fourth, and in one case the fifth test came back positive. The tests were repeated at 1- to 3-day intervals (Li et al., 2020).

In our patient, the sample was sent again on Day 8 of the illness. RT-PCR for SARS-COV2 again came back negative. His condition didn't improve.

Q2) What to do after repeat RT-PCR came back negative?

Ultimately, on Day 10, bronchoscopy was done to obtain a sample from the lower airway. A BAL (bronchoalveolar lavage) fluid was sent for RT-PCR. It came back positive for SARS-COV2.

The above cases illustrate that despite having multiple guidelines, at times it is the clinician who will have to take the call depending on the situation at hand.

THE GLOBAL CHALLENGE

When the epidemic unfolded globally in early 2020, most of the countries were taken unawares. After the standardized tests were developed, most countries tried to develop their own testing strategies. Testing was important in order to confirm the cases, isolate them, and trace the contacts to prevent further spread of the disease. The **test positivity rate** (number of tests coming back positive divided by the number of tests done) provided an objective measure of how adequately countries were testing. It also gave an idea about how the virus spread. According to the WHO, **a test positive rate of less than 5%** is one indicator that the epidemic is under control in a country (WHO, May 2020) (Figure 7.5).

Different countries chose to follow different paths depending on their past experience, resources at hand, and the decision-making

The share of COVID-19 tests that are positive

The daily positive rate, given as a rolling 7-day average.

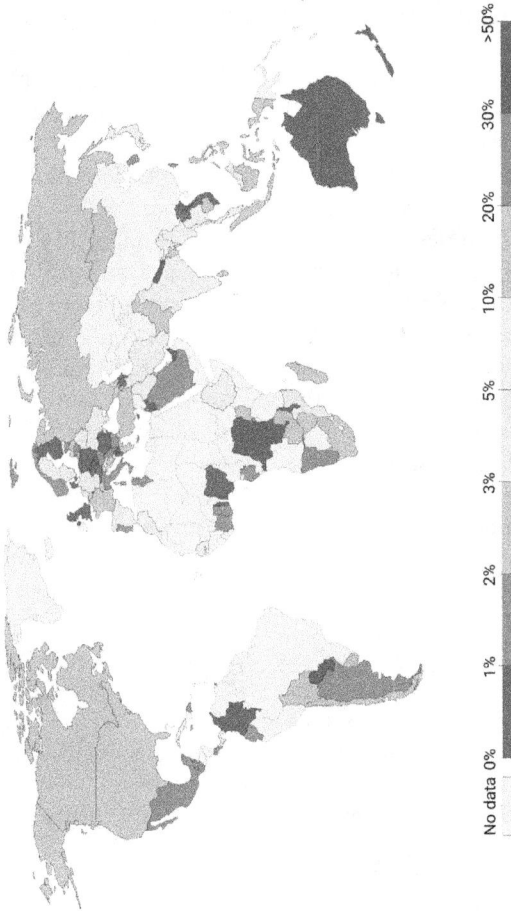

| No data | 0% | 1% | 2% | 3% | 5% | 10% | 20% | 30% | >50% |

Source: Official data collated by Our World in Data – Last updated 11 June, 13:30 (London time)   OurWorldInData.org/coronavirus • CC BY
Note: Comparisons of testing data across countries are affected by differences in the way the data are reported. Daily data is interpolated for countries not reporting testing data on a daily basis. Details can be found at our Testing Dataset page

Figure 7.5 Test positive rate

process. Some countries like South Korea seemed to have learnt from their past flawed response to a MERS outbreak of 2015, and they built infection control staff and isolation units, expanded outbreak simulations and PPE training, and started community-based collaboration between medical centres and local governments. South Korea already had 12.3 beds per 1,000 population (one of the highest in the world). Once the pandemic started, they quickly ramped up their testing capacity and made it widely available. By April 2020, the testing capacity increased to 20,000 per day and in November 2020, the capacity reached 110,000 per day (Kim et al, 2021).

This early, adequate testing led to a quick control of the pandemic with decline in the number of cases by mid-March.

In some countries, wide free testing is still not available (Figure 7.6).

In some countries like Russia and Brazil testing policy is yet to be clearly delineated. Along with test positive rates, the **number of tests done per confirmed case** is a sensitive indicator of the test adequacy (the WHO suggesting at least 10 to 20 tests per confirmed case).

On the other hand, some countries like the United Kingdom chose to test judiciously only the affected individuals from high-risk groups. This was done with a view that any "suspected" patient needs to be kept in isolation. They were to be hospitalized and tested only if they were symptomatic. This point of view was taken in order to prudently use the limited testing resources and prevent overwhelming of the hospital capacities. Inadequate testing led to significantly more affected individuals than confirmed cases. Contact tracing also failed.

Italy, on 1 April, 2020, had one confirmed case for every 5 to 10 tests. The number of cases increased and overwhelmed the existing health infrastructure. Italy soon ramped its testing capacity, and on 1.6.20, it was testing 100 people per positive case (Hasell et al., 2021).

What became more and more evident was that while in short term "priority testing" may conserve resources, long-term expansion of the testing facility was imperative. A widely available testing facility was key to achieve control of the situation by isolating patients and identifying their contacts.

Just increasing the testing capacity was only one factor. The other factor was the timing of the increase. The United States, after the initial delay in March, started extensive testing in April and May. But by then the pandemic had spread as evident from the view from New York (Mukherjee et al., 2022).

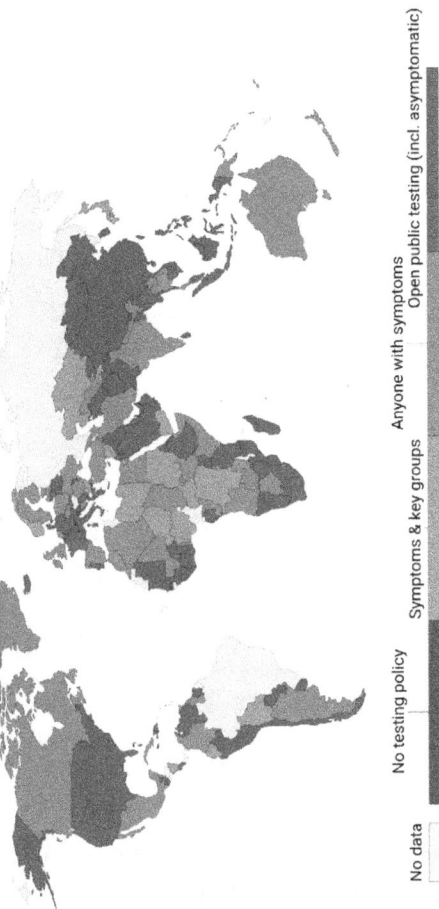

COVID-19 Testing Policies, Jun 13, 2021

– No testing policy.
– Only those who both (a) have symptoms and also (b) meet specific criteria (e.g. key workers, admitted to hospital, came into contact with a known case, returned from overseas).
– Testing of anyone showing COVID-19 symptoms.
– Open public testing (e.g. "drive through" testing available to asymptomatic people).

No data | No testing policy | Symptoms & key groups | Anyone with symptoms | Open public testing (incl. asymptomatic)

Source: Hale, Angrist, Goldszmidt, Kira, Petherick, Phillips, Webster, Cameron-Blake, Hallas, Majumdar, and Tatlow (2021). "A global panel database of pandemic policies (Oxford COVID-19 Government Response Tracker)." Nature Human Behaviour. – Last updated 13 June. 06.17 (London time)
OurWorldInData.org/coronavirus • CC BY

Figure 7.6 Testing policy in COVID-19 patients

Apart from testing adequately and testing early, the third factor that comes to play is the **contact tracing**. South Korea employed personal information like credit card, security footage, and phone data to do a thorough and extensive contact tracing. This made the testing protocol more fruitful and effective. Apart from manual interview, an important advancement was app-based contact tracing. Singapore was one of the first countries to roll out the *Trace Together* app. India's *Aarogyo Setu* app was also developed for the purpose of instant contact tracing in real time. Ghosh et al. (2020) also notes that in Thailand one main reason for lower incidence of the pandemic in the first wave was the presence of a million volunteers who were mobilized after the SARS outbreak.

However, data privacy issues might be hampering wide-scale adoption of many of the apps which might be addressed to some extent by instituting some sunset clauses as proposed by academics at Singapore Management University (Tham and Loke, 2020).

INDIA

India faced numerous challenges at the start of the pandemic. It had a population of roughly 1,400 million. The economic resources were limited, but the density of population extremely high (423.88 people/sq Km), especially in urban centres. India had 0.55 hospital beds in government capacity per 1,000 population. The % of GDP being spent by the government on healthcare was extremely low (1.6%) (Ghosh et al., 2022).

In India, direct reliable tests like RT-PCR for SARS-COV2 could be done in only few centres like the National Institute of Virology, Pune. The Government of India under Prime Minister Narendra Modi ordered a nationwide lockdown on 24 March 2020 for 21 days. This was later extended till 31 May 2020 in a desperate effort to slow down the spread of COVID-19. In the meantime, both the central government and the state governments, along with leading private labs, soon started to expand the testing potential (Chatterjee, 2022). Even PPEs were in shortage from less than 10,000 tests per day in March, to more than a million samples in June; testing capacity was expanded at breakneck pace with sufficient quality control and state supervision. However, this was still not adequate as the infection had spread by then.

There was some variability regarding the nature of tests being performed by the various states. While some states like Tamil Nadu relied exclusively on the RT-PCR testing method to determine their cases, some states like Maharashtra used a combination of RT-PCR and RATs. Some states like Uttar Pradesh, Kerala, Gujarat, and Bihar seemed to rely more on the RATs (>50% of the tests) for their case detection. RATs had lower sensitivity compared to RT-PCR, but had a quicker TAT. This led to non-uniformity in data.

In March 2020, when the outbreak started, testing was allowed in a government lab free of cost for only those with history of recent international travel and having symptoms or those who had come in contact with a laboratory-confirmed COVID-19 patient or healthcare workers who were managing SARI and were symptomatic. The private labs could do the test only on advice of a qualified physician as per ICMR protocol. Later, the testing indications were slowly expanded.

The first wave subsided towards the winter of 2020, but returned in an even more infectious and virulent form in the spring of 2021. This second wave may have been caused by the mutant strains, poor mask compliance, overcrowding, and a lowering of the immunity level beyond 6 months.

This time the lab infrastructure was better prepared. India had 2,506 molecular testing laboratories with a National Testing capacity of 1.5 million tests per day considering a three-shift operationalization. But still the unprecedented surge of cases overwhelmed the operational capacity.

The ICMR suggested measures to optimize the RT-PCR testing and simultaneously increase the access and availability of testing to all citizens of the country. (Reference ICMR bulletin 4.5.21)

i   RT-PCR test must not be repeated in any individual who has tested positive once either by RAT or RT-PCR.

ii   No testing is required for COVID-19-recovered individuals at the time of hospital discharge.

iii   The need for RT-PCR test in healthy individuals undertaking inter-state domestic travel may be completely removed to reduce the load on laboratories.

iv   Non-essential travel and interstate travel of symptomatic individuals (COVID-19 or flulike symptoms) should be essentially avoided.

v   Mobile testing laboratories are now available on the GeM portal.

RATs are recommended in India for COVID-19 testing in June 2020. However, the use of these tests is mainly limited to containment zones and healthcare settings. The ICMR suggested making these tests more accessible due to their advantage of short TAT.

The Indian response to the pandemic has had to make pragmatic compromises. Decades of inadequate investment and lack of development of adequate health infrastructure has led to several shortcomings in the testing procedure. This has been more evident in the rural areas. The healthcare personnel worked 24/7 to ensure maximum utilization of the testing capacity. There have been successes like in Dharavi (the largest slum in Mumbai) where POC testing led to rapid control of the outbreak.

Only testing is not enough. Adequate contact tracing is a must. This is virtually impossible in the crowded Indian cities. Social distancing and proper use of masks also need to be overemphasized. Otherwise, subsequent waves of the pandemic will continue to come back till adequate herd immunity is reached through vaccination in 2022.

CONCLUSION

This pandemic has been an eye opener in more ways than one. For the microbiologists, it has shown that newer microbes are going to challenge human existence. As humans encroach on animal habitats disrespecting the barriers of nature with disdain, species jumping can threaten our very existence.

Molecular biology has to rise to this challenge and make more sensitive, specific tests available at a lower cost. POC tests of nucleic acids that can be done faster is still evolving. The main challenge has been to get these tests done in the community set-up. Antigen tests are still being standardized. The clinician should be the person decide what test to do. A sensitive antigen test which can be self-administered using a saliva specimen is yet to come.

At the level of the policymakers, this has been more of a learning process. Prior preparation has been the key to success in controlling this pandemic. The countries who had prior preparation performed well. The earlier one can detect, the better it is. Co-operation should be sought from the public by the government. Under-the-skin surveillance will face resistance. Global cooperation and sharing of information is important as more and more mutants crop up (Ghosh et al., 2022). This is needed not only for sharing of data but also for ramping up test facilities and health infrastructure.

> If we choose global solidarity, it will be a victory not only against the coronavirus, but against all future epidemics and crises that might assail humankind in the 21st century.
>
> (Yuval Noah Harari, 2020)

NOTE

This contributed chapter was accepted for publication in this refereed edited volume on June 20, 2021.

REFERENCES

Ansede, M., A. Galocha, M. Zafra, (2020), "CCU CGG CGG GCA the 12 letters that changed the world." Consulte la Portada de EL PAIS Edicion Nacional del 3 de Octubre.

Basu, M., (2020), "RT-PCR, antigen, antibody, TrueNAT — all you need to know about the different Covid tests." *The Print*, 27 June, 2020, https://theprint.in/science/rt-pcr-antigen-antibody-truenat-all-you-need-to-know-about-the-different-covid-tests/448733/ (27 June, 2020).

Binnicker, M. J., (2020), "Challenges and controversies to testing for COVID-19." *Journal of Clinical Microbiology*, 58:11, pp. e0 1695–20.

Biswas, S., K. Pathi, (2020), "India's new paper Covid-19 test could be a 'game changer,'" 5 October 2020, https://www.bbc.com/news/world-asia-india-54338864.

Bollineni, V. R. et al., (2021), "The role of CT imaging for management of COVID-19 in epidemic area: early experience from a University Hospital Insights Imaging," 12:10. doi:10.1186/s13244-020-00957-5.

Cascella, M, M. Rajnik, A. Cuomo, S. C. Dulebohn, R. Di Napoli, (2020), "Features, evaluation and treatment coronavirus (COVID-19)." *StatPearls* [Internet]. StatPearls Publishing.

Centers for Disease Control and Prevention (CDC), (2020), "Overview of testing for SARS-CoV2 (COVID-19)" [cited 15 December 2020] In: CDC website. Atlanta, GA.

Chatterjee, S., (2022), "Virtual Fireside Conversations with Business Leaders," In *Managing Complexity and Covid19: Life, Liberty or The Pursuit of Happiness*, Editors A. Ghosh, A. Haldar and K. Bhaumik. Routledge, pp. 150–154.

Chong, C., (2021), "Rapid tests to be used in S'pore on top of PCR tests for quicker Covid-19 contact tracing." https://www.straitstimes.com/singapore/rapid-tests-to-be-used-in-spore-on-top-of-pcr-tests-for-quicker-contact-tracing-and, June 3, 2021.

Corman, V. M., O. Landt, M. Kaiser, R. Molenkamp, A. Meijer, D. K. Chu, (2020), "Detection of 2019 novel coronavirus (2019-nCoV) by real-time RT-PCR." *Euro Surveill.* doi:10.2807/1560-7917.ES.2020.25.3.2000045.

Fredericks, D. N., D. A., Relman, (1996), "Sequence-based identification of microbial pathogens: a reconsideration of Koch's postulates." *Clinical Microbiology Reviews*, Jan. 1996; 9:1, pp. 18–33.

Ghosh, A., (2022), "Strategic debate on financial inclusion: is life or livelihood a false choice." In *Managing Complexity and Covid19: Life, Liberty, or the Pursuit of Happiness*, Editors A. Ghosh, A. Haldar and K. Bhaumik. Routledge, pp. 3–19.

Ghosh A., et al., (2022), "COVID-19 herd immunity and role of vaccines." In *Managing Complexity and Covid19: Life, Liberty, or the Pursuit of Happiness*, Editors A. Ghosh, A. Haldar and K. Bhaumik. Routledge, pp. 130–144.

Ghosh, A., W.-K., Lim, A. Haldar, K. Bhaumik, (2020), "The Covid-19 crisis in Thailand: charting a safe and sustainable path to recovery." Case No: SMU-20–0041, CMP, Singapore Management University, Singapore.

Green, A., (2020), "Li Wenliang." *Lancet*, 395:10225, p. 682.

Guo, L., L. Ren, S. Yang, et al. (2020), "Profiling early humoral response to diagnose novel coronavirus disease (COVID-19)." *Clinical Infectious Diseases*; ciaa310. Published online March 21, 2020. doi:10.1093/cid/ciaa310.

Harari, Y. N., (2020), "The world after coronavirus." *Financial Times*, March 20, 2020.

Hasell, J., (2021), "Testing early, testing late: four countries' approaches to COVID-19 testing compared." https://ourworldindata.org/covid-testing-us-uk-korea-italy.

Hoffmann, M., H. Kleine-Weber, S. Schroeder, N. Krüger, T. Herrler, S. Erichsen, et al., (2020), "SARS-CoV-2 cell entry depends on ACE2 and TMPRSS2 and is blocked by a clinically proven protease inhibitor." *Cell.* doi:10.1016/j.cell.2020.02.052.

ICMR guidelines 19.5.21. "Advisory for COVID-19 Home Testing using Rapid Antigen Tests (RATs)." https://www.icmr.gov.in

Kim, J.-H., et al., "Emerging COVID-19 success story: South Korea learned the lessons of MERS2021." https://ourworldindata.org/covid-exemplar-south-korea.

Li, Y., et al. (2020), "Stability issues of RT-PCR testing of SARS-CoV2 for hospitalized patients with clinically diagnosed with COVID-19." *Journal of Medical Virology*, 92:7, pp. 903–908.

Mousavizadeh, L., S. Ghasemi, (2020), "Genotype and phenotype of COVID-19: their roles in pathogenesis." *Journal of Microbiology, Immunology and Infection.* doi:10.1016/j.jmii.2020.03.022.

Mukherjee, V., et al. (2022), "View from the frontline." In *Managing Complexity and Covid19: Life, Liberty, or the Pursuit of Happiness*, Editors A. Ghosh, A. Haldar and K. Bhaumik. Routledge, pp. 121–129.

See, S., (2021), "30 fully vaccinated individuals test positive for Covid-19, with mild to no symptoms: Gan Kim Yong." https://www.businesstimes.com.sg/government-economy/30-fully-vaccinated-individuals-test-positive-for-covid-19-with-mild-to-no." June 6, 2021.

Sethuraman, N., S. Sunderaraj, R. Akhide, (2020), "Interpreting diagnostic tests for Sars-CoV2." *JAMA*, 323:22, pp. 2249–2251.

Statnews, (2020), "WHO comments on asymptomatic spread of Covid-19." https://www.statnews.com/2020/06/09/who-comments-asymptomatic-spread-covid-19/, June 17, 2020.

Stephanie, S., S. Thomas, et al. (2020), "Determinants of chest radiography sensitivity for Covid 19: a multi-institutional study in the United States." *Radiology: Cardiothoracic Imaging*, 2:5, p. e200337.

Tham, B., J. Y. Loke, (2020), "Sunset clause for contact tracing apps could build trust and aid wider adoption," https://www.straitstimes.com/opinion/sunset-clause-for-contact-tracing-apps-could-build-trust-and-aid-wider-adoption, June 17, 2020.

Wang, W., Y. Xu, R. Gao, et al. (2020), "Detection of SARS-CoV-2 in different types of clinical specimens." *JAMA*, Published online March 11, 2020. doi:10. 1001/jama.2020.3786.

WHO, (2020), Public health criteria to adjust public health and social measures in the context of COVID-19, 12 May 2020.

Zhao, J., Q. Yuan, H. Wang, et al., (2020), "Antibody responses to SARS CoV-2 in patients of novel coronavirus disease 2019." *Clinical Infectious Diseases*, Nov 19, 71:16, pp. 2027–2034.

8

THE EFFICACY OF MASK MANDATES IN THE UNITED STATES DURING THE EARLY DAYS OF THE PANDEMIC

Rajesh Ranjan Nandy

INTRODUCTION

In the early days of the pandemic, there was no global consensus on the efficacy of mask usage towards controlling the spread of the COVID-19 virus. In fact, in the United States, the Centre for Disease Control recommended against wearing masks for healthy people as a protection against respiratory illness from COVID-19 (Feng et al., 2020). However, as COVID-19 started to spread globally, there has been growing evidence in favour of wearing masks for infected people (both symptomatic and asymptomatic) towards controlling the spread of the COVID-19 virus. Global organizations, such as the World Health Organizations, have started to modify their initial recommendations on wearing masks, from recommending against it to more usage of it (World Health Organization 2020). In the end, the scientific community reached a broad consensus on the efficacy of mask usage in public settings in controlling the pandemic. However, in the United States, in spite of a general agreement among policymakers on the efficacy of masks, there has been a raging debate on actually issuing an official mandate on mask usage at public places instead of simply recommending the usage (Lyu and Wehby, 2020). Many policymakers have been in favour of relying on retailers and other businesses to

DOI: 10.4324/9781003218807-10

come up with their own policies on wearing of masks. Due to a lack of consensus on the issuance of mask mandates, there was no universal policy across the nation, in the early days of the pandemic. Instead, different states had different policies, and even within the same state, different counties and cities had different official policies on mask usage. In this chapter, we investigate the actual effect of mask mandates in the early days of the pandemic using three different approaches. First, we will look at the county-level COVID-19 daily case data across the United States, among the counties most affected in the early days and compare the basic reproduction ratios (R_0) among the counties with or without a mandate. Next, we will assess the efficacy of early intervention in issuing a mask mandate from a prevention perspective, using state-level data in the 50 states and the District of Columbia (DC) in the United States. Finally, we will assess the efficacy of late intervention from a reversal of trend perspective by using county-level data in the greater Dallas metropolitan.

METHODS AND RESULTS

In the first approach, in studying the efficacy of mask mandates, we considered 147 counties across the United States with a total number of reported cases of over 2,500 (as of June 17, 2020). For each of these counties, we tracked the daily occurrence of new reported cases since the onset of the pandemic. The data on daily reported new cases were collected from the Johns Hopkins Coronavirus Resource Centre (2020). To account for a cyclic weekly variation, a seven-day moving average of the number of daily new reported cases was used for our analysis. Using the smoothed data, we estimated the R_0 for each county. We then compared the R_0 values (as of June 17, 2020) for the counties where a mandate had been issued with the counties where no mandate had been issued. In Figure 8.1, we plotted the overlaying histograms of R_0 values of counties with a mask mandate (green) and counties without a mask mandate (red). The mean R_0 in counties with no mandate are 1.0595298 as opposed to 0.8223954 for counties with a mandate on usage of masks in public places. The difference in R_0 is highly significant statistically with a p-value of 4.778×10^{-14}.

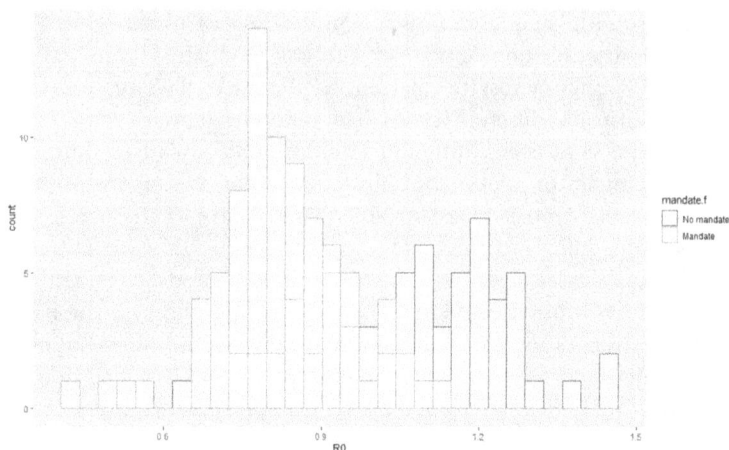

Figure 8.1 Histograms for counties in the United States with and without mandates on masks

To assess the efficacy of early intervention from a prevention perspective, we noted that nationally in the United States, the initial wave peaked in April, followed by a slow decline till the end of May, with a surge in late June. We have identified 14 states (CT, DE, DC, HI, IL, MA, MD, ME, NM, NJ, NY, PA, RI, VA), where an early mandate was issued by May before the surge in June. We compared the growth in average number of daily cases between end of May and mid-July 2020 between these states with early mandate and the rest of the states without an early state-wide mandate. For each of the 50 states and DC, we first calculated the average number of daily new cases per 100,000 population in the last week of May and the week ending in July 18. We then compared the change in average number of daily new cases per 100,000 population between the states with and without state-wide mandates. Statistically, the results are highly significant with states without a mandate exhibiting on average an increase of 14 daily new cases per 100,000 population as opposed to a decrease in 2.5 daily new cases per 100,000 population for states with a mandate (p-value 1.46×10^{-5}). In the visual representation in Figure 8.2, we plotted the change in average number of daily new cases per 100,000 population in each of the 50 states and DC. For all the states with a mask mandate effective in May, there is

50 States and District of Columbia

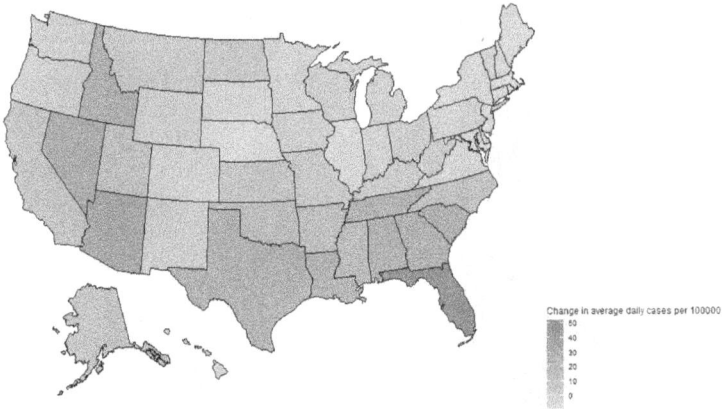

Change in average daily cases per 100000
- 50
- 40
- 30
- 20
- 10
- 0

Figure 8.2 The change in average number of daily new cases per 100,000 population in each of the 50 states and DC

either a decrease in the average number of daily new cases (CT, DE, DC, IL, MA, MD, ME, NJ, NY, RI, VA) or a marginal increase (HI, NM, PA). For the states without a mask mandate effective in May, only three states (NE, NH, and SD) exhibit a decrease in the average number of daily new cases, and each of these three states is sparsely populated. The remaining 34 states without mask mandate exhibit an increase in the average number of daily new cases. Furthermore, all the states with the largest increase in the average number of adjusted daily new cases are those without mask mandate in May.

Finally, in our third approach, we assess the efficacy of the late issuance of mandates in controlling the June surge. Once the surge in the number of new cases across the nation became apparent in mid-June, issuance of mask mandates had been more prevalent at city, county, and state levels. However, due to the lag in the appearance of symptoms after infection, testing, and reporting, any impact of a new policy on the transmission of the disease is only apparent after approximately 10–14 days. Since the local and state mandates had been issued over an extended period, beginning in the third week of June, a comprehensive nationwide study on the efficacy of these late mandates is beyond the scope of this chapter. Instead, we

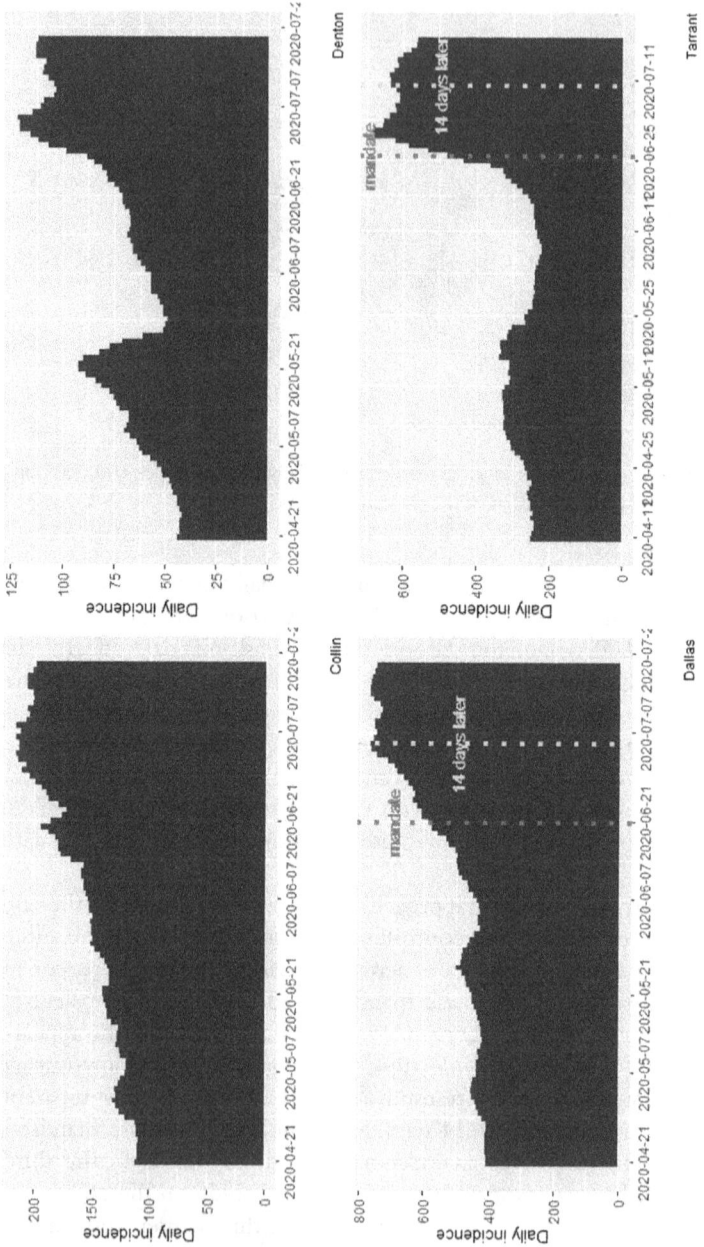

Figure 8.3 The daily incidence

will study the efficacy of the local mandates in the two largest counties (Dallas and Tarrant) in the Dallas metropolitan area, towards reversing the trend. We have comprehensive data available from these two counties to reach a meaningful conclusion. It should be noted that daily reported positive COVID-19 case counts pose a statistical challenge, as there is a lag in getting infected and showing symptoms to get tested. There is a further lag in getting a confirmation of the test. Both lags are random in nature. Also, there may be a lag in reporting the positive test result, resulting in unusually low or high case counts on certain days. To mitigate these effects, we used the suspected number of COVID-19-related illness, leading to an ER visit in the last 24 hours as a proxy for the number of new cases in any given day. This has the advantage of the number being less susceptible to lack of proper testing and inaccurate reporting dates of actual cases. For a more precise estimation of R_0, we simply needed to assume that the number of new ER visits is proportional to the true number of new COVID-19 infections of each day. The ER visits data for suspected COVID patients were made available by North Central Texas Trauma Regional Advisory Council (NCT-TRAC). We plotted the daily incidences of suspected COVID-19-related illness leading to an ER visit (Figure 8.3) and then estimated the trend in the time varying R_0 for these two counties. A reversal in the trend is quite apparent in both Dallas and Tarrant Counties in the expected timeframe based on mask mandate, with Tarrant County depicting a sharp change.

DISCUSSION

There has been a raging debate across the globe and more specifically in the United States in terms of the right policies and mitigating measures in controlling the spread of coronavirus. Every conceivable proposal to contain the spread has certain trade-offs. On one end of the spectrum, the policy demands closure of schools and nonessential businesses as well as shelter-in-place orders. However, such a policy puts enormous burden on the local economy and broad societal health (as evidenced by more incidences of obesity, diminished student learning, loss of jobs, etc.). Hence, an extreme policy can be implemented only in the short run, as a last resort. At the other end of the spectrum, there is effectively no enforceable policy except for general recommendations on wearing masks and maintaining social distancing as well as personal hygiene. This policy has the least economic burden but is least effective in controlling the spread, and has the potential risk of a high death toll. In our opinion, mandating a strong mask usage policy with moderate restrictions on economic activities can be an ideal middle ground with low economic burden. Using three different approaches, we have provided strong evidence that a mask mandate can effectively control the spread of the disease without an overly restrictive shelter-in-place order. It should be noted that the differences observed in each of these cases is quite significant. Specifically, in our comparison of R_0 among counties with or without mask mandates, we observed an estimated difference of 0.24. Due to the exponential nature of transmission, a reduction of 0.24 in R_0 can potentially prevent thousands of new cases and subsequent deaths.

Masks and face coverings are simple and inexpensive. For most healthy people, the only real price of wearing a mask is minor inconvenience. There may be some additional auxiliary benefits of wearing masks, in terms of protection from various forms of allergies and germs. In fact, the extremely low nationwide cases of the flu this year can partly be attributed to the wearing of masks. We consider the failure to universally recommend or mandate the usage of mask in public places in the early days of the pandemic to be truly unfortunate as it could have significantly reduced the death toll.

LIMITATIONS

First and foremost, what we have clearly demonstrated is a strong association between mask mandates and controlling the spread of the virus. However, association does not necessarily imply causation. But the preponderance of evidence and the trend indeed suggests causation even if it cannot be proven conclusively.

Next, the exact nature of the mandate is not homogeneous across the nation, and there may be other mitigating measures or factors not considered in the analysis (such as compliance with other social distancing measures, workforce distribution, population density, population demographic, socioeconomic, and cultural factors).

In our comparison of states with or without a state-wide mandate, it should be noted that our analysis is purely based on state mandates. Many cities and counties had local mandates in effect, and the impact of the local mandates is not captured in the analysis. Furthermore, issuance of mandate does not necessarily imply compliance, and we do not have data currently available to adjust for actual compliance. Nonetheless, the observed effect is large enough to conclude, with confidence, that the overall impact of early mask mandates has been positive in preventing a surge in most of the states with a state-wide mandate.

It should also be noted that our findings are relevant for the early days of the pandemic when there is a lack of overall awareness among the population about the disease. In the later days of the pandemic, the mandate may not have played such a big role after the rollout of vaccination. In fact, in the state of Texas, no noticeable change in trend was observed after the mask mandate was lifted.

Finally, it is possible that when the spread of infection grows alarmingly high in a specific region, people are more compliant with the recommended guidelines of mask wearing and other measures. This may serve as a potential confounding for the efficacy of the mandate.

CONCLUSIONS

Despite the stated limitations, the data strongly suggest that a mask mandate is highly effective in controlling the spread of the virus. Until herd immunity from COVID-19 is achieved through a combination of vaccination and recovery from infection, the usage of mask is highly recommended.

NOTE

This contributed chapter was accepted for publication in this refereed edited volume on June 28, 2021.

REFERENCES

John Hopkins Coronavirus Resource Centre. United States cases by county. Johns Hopkins University & Medicine. Retrieved July 15, 2020, from https://coronavirus.jhu.edu/.

Feng S, Shen C, Xia N, Song W, Fan M, Cowling BJ. Rational use of face masks in the COVID-19 pandemic. Lancet Respir Med. 2020;8(5):434–6.

Lyu W, Wehby GL. Community use of face masks and COVID-19: evidence from a natural experiment of state mandates in the US. Health Aff (Millwood). 2020 Aug;39(8):1419–25. doi:10.1377/hlthaff.2020.00818. Epub 2020 Jun 16. PMID: 32543923.

World Health Organization. (2020). Advice on the use of masks in the context of COVID-19: interim guidance, 6 April 2020. World Health Organization. https://apps.who.int/iris/handle/10665/331693. License: CC BY-NC-SA 3.0 IGO.

9

VIEW FROM THE FRONTLINE: NEW YORK CITY[1]

Vikramjit Mukherjee, Himanshu Deshwal, and Alok Bhatt

NEW YORK CITY—A VIEW FROM THE FRONTLINES

New York City is a sprawling metropolis with a population of 8.3 million (U.S. Census Bureau, 2021), encompassing an extremely broad socioeconomic spectrum. Approximately 42.7% of the population identifies as white, 24.3% as black or African American, and 13.9% as Asian. In 2018, the median household income was $60,762 and the per capita income was $37,693. 18.9% of persons were identified as living in poverty. In comparison, the median monthly rent was $1,396, representing 44% of total per capita income (New York State Department of Health).

There is significant economic disparity among the five boroughs of the city, with the median income in Manhattan being more than twice the median income in the Bronx (New York State Department of Health). This disparity is evident in other health indicators as well, with Manhattan and Staten Island having the highest rates of health insurance among adults aged 18–64 (~93% in 2016) compared to the Bronx and Queens (~87% in 2016). Additionally, healthcare utilization through emergency department visits is significantly higher in the Bronx (age-adjusted rate 6,757.7 per 10,000 persons) compared to Manhattan (4,158.1) or Queens (3,846).

DOI: 10.4324/9781003218807-11

Hospitalization rates also demonstrate the same pattern. Other indicators, like access to regular healthcare and food security, also vary by county.

There are many reasons for these variations including, but not limited to, the nature of each borough's residents (immigration status, ethnicity, English as a spoken language, nature of employment, among others). Manhattan is the administrative and financial centre of the city, attracting highly skilled workers that work in finance, healthcare, and entertainment industries. On the other hand, Queens is home to the most ethnically diverse urban neighbourhoods in the United States (O'Donnell, 2006), as well as the world (Weber, 2013).

A city like New York has unique features that are essential to its daily function, which possibly served to amplify outbreaks of disease, as seen during the COVID-19 pandemic. Manhattan has a high population density of 27,544 persons/km^2, compared to 8,018 persons/km^2 in Queens. However, Queens averages 3 persons per household, compared to Manhattan where people are crowded in small, yet separate apartments, inside high-rise buildings averaging 2 persons per household. Additionally, an estimated 44% of the population in Queens is foreign born, and these residents live in close-knit communities that frequently gather in numbers, owing to tradition and culture.

The New York City (NYC) Subway is the busiest rapid transit system in the Western World, and the ninth busiest rapid transit rail system in the world (Web.mta.info, 2021), with an annual subway ridership of 1.75 billion. Many busy lines on this subway operate beyond capacity, and overcrowding is common both at stations and inside subway cars, leading to prolonged air recirculation in a closed space.

In addition to local factors, NYC also has the busiest airport system in the United States, with over 140 million passengers passing through the various airports under the authority of the Port Authority Aviation Department (Port Authority NYNJ). JFK airport alone accounted for 6.26 million of these air passengers. This served as a large catchment for incoming international travellers who could import any number of infectious diseases. All these factors played a significant role in making NYC the centre of this pandemic in early Spring, 2020.

THE SURGE

The first confirmed case of COVID-19 in the United States was reported on January 21, 2020; the WHO declared a global health emergency on 30 January 2020. On 1 March 2020, NYC reported its first case. As the number of positive cases rose, the Department of Health and Mental Hygiene (DOHMH) issued comprehensive guidance on testing, quarantine, and isolation. Asymptomatic individuals who had been exposed to a case (person with a positive COVID-19 test) were advised to quarantine for a period of 14 days after their last exposure (NYC Health, 2021). New York University and a handful of other institutions were the first to implement a ban on all business-related travel. Soon, other institutions and state governments followed suit with stringent guidelines advising against all non-essential travel, and quarantine upon traveling between states.

There were issues with testing that precluded effective tracing of cases and contacts. The US Centre for Disease Control and Prevention had to withdraw testing kits in March 2020 when they were shown to have a high rate of false-positives due to reagent contamination (Willman, 2020). Restrictions by the federal government on testing by individual states lasted until early March. As cases in NYC increased exponentially, the city announced restrictions on testing of non-hospitalized persons to prevent crowding of hospitals by persons seeking to get themselves tested. This was done with the intent to reduce person-to-person spread by patients seeking out testing for milder symptoms. At the same time, a nationwide shortage of testing reagents further imposed limitations on both, the number of tests that could be performed, as well as the turnaround time for results (Cuza, 2020). As institutions were finally able to implement in-house testing, problems with more rapid tests started to become apparent, with faster results achieved at the high cost of significantly reduced accuracy (Basu et al., 2020). Furthermore, the extremely high community prevalence of the disease often meant that negative results did not change the management of patients presenting with respiratory symptoms. The absence of reliable testing strategies with quick turnaround time crippled public health measures to identify, trace, and isolate people who were exposed to SARS-CoV-2 virus-infected persons.

By early April, NYC was seeing upwards of 10,000 new cases every day. Early epidemiologic modelling estimated that within two weeks all hospital beds would be occupied, and there would be a shortage of ventilators by several thousands. The boroughs of Brooklyn and Queens were disproportionately affected, and the local hospitals were quickly overrun. This led to significant stress on the healthcare system, with consequences on patient outcomes. While initial reports from China had suggested features of severe respiratory distress syndrome as the clinical presentation, in NYC the experience included many more complications. Patients experienced multiple organ failure, including renal failure that required urgent dialysis. There were many incidents of large clots in various organs, such as the lungs, heart, limbs, and brain, causing sudden deaths. The medical community was now in hitherto unknown territory. Several longitudinal, prospective studies are being conducted to assess the long-term mental and physical impact of the disease in COVID-19 survivors who were admitted to the intensive care unit (ICU) for respiratory failure.

THE RESPONSE

On 7 March 2020, New York Governor Andrew Cuomo declared a state of emergency, and several restrictions on transportation, gatherings, and social events were imposed to contain the spread of COVID-19. By 13 March 2020, a national emergency was declared, and the bustling city of New York came to a standstill. At Bellevue Hospital, as is likely with many others, most hospital rooms were rapidly converted into negative-pressure rooms (a form of air ventilation in hospital rooms required for air-borne pathogens such as tuberculosis, influenza, or SARS-CoV-2) as hospitals restructured to care for COVID-19 patients. Health systems quickly began to be stretched to their limits with the volume of patient influx. ICUs were especially hard hit owing to the level of care required for each patient.

The expected shortage of ventilators was partially addressed by the arrival of emergency ventilators supplied by the Federal Emergency Management Agency (FEMA). However, other resources including haemodialysis machines, and more importantly, medical staff, remained inadequate in the early stages. But shortages were answered through innovation. For example, the number of patients experiencing acute renal failure took us by surprise and exceeded the available haemodialysis machines and nurses. Peritoneal dialysis, which does not require a haemodialysis machine or intensive nurse staffing and is a well-established mode of dialysis in end-stage renal disease patients, helped reserve haemodialysis machines for sicker and new patients who needed them more.

The volume of patient influx during the surge in the city was extraordinary. In response, hundreds of nurses, physicians, and respiratory therapists from different parts of the country that were as yet relatively unaffected volunteered to join the fight in New York. Their contribution and commitment reflected the solidarity of the medical community, and their inexhaustible willingness to care for patients, even at the risk of their own safety.

The community played a significant role in supporting healthcare workers. Many individuals and non-profit organizations donated money to sponsor meals for healthcare workers. People donated their previously stockpiled personal protective equipment (PPE) to hospitals and healthcare workers. Every day at 7 PM shift change, the people of NYC cheered all the healthcare providers on, from their balcony.

HEALTHCARE WORKER PERSPECTIVE

We listened carefully to narratives from the frontlines in China during the initial phase of the pandemic, hoping for insight into our upcoming fight. While preparations were extensive, NYC was affected like no other city in the world. As critical care physicians, we were ready for the challenge, but there remained a lurking fear of the unknown. No validated treatment strategy had yet been established, and strategies were only anecdotal. When the surge came, it hit medical community hard, fast, and in multiple deadly waves. Every day we admitted several patients with severe multi-organ dysfunction. COVID-19 did not distinguish between young or old, healthy or frail. We watched patients in their early twenties and in their late eighties die despite our best efforts to treat and revive them. Their lungs were severely damaged. Some developed sudden blood clots cutting off supply to vital organs, which could not be restored. Due to strict isolation policies, family members could not visit their loved ones, and communication was over the phone. Watching our best efforts fail and conveying bad news to families took a significant emotional toll on all those working on the frontlines. Many workers separated themselves from their families and children to protect them from getting infected. Several moved into a hotel or sent their families away to grandparents or relatives to isolate, not seeing them again for weeks or months. Working anywhere between 12 and 18 hours a day, all we could think about is how to save the next patient.

The pandemic was not without success stories that rejuvenated our belief and courage to keep fighting and keep caring for the sick. We found ourselves learning about a new disease at an unbelievable pace. Studying the physiologic response to the SARS-CoV-2 virus was an excellent academic opportunity. Those training in critical care obtained the kind of experience that would otherwise take several years to accumulate. In many ways, we were able to overcome our fear and exhaustion with excitement and in some cases, a sense of achievement. There was a certain exhilaration when we wheeled patients out of the hospital to be discharged; patients who days or weeks ago were fighting for their lives on life support.

One such story is that of a young 18-year-old woman who was 35 weeks pregnant when she was admitted with symptoms of COVID-19. Her clinical status took a turn for the worse and her oxygen saturation started to drop rapidly. The chest radiograph was concerning for acute respiratory distress syndrome. In this case, it was not just one, but two lives at stake. Along with our obstetrics team, we decided to put the patient on a mechanical ventilator and perform an urgent caesarean section to deliver the baby in a negative-pressure operating room. The surgery was successful, and a healthy baby boy was born. The mother remained on ventilator support initially but was successfully taken off the ventilator and sent to the obstetrics floor after three days. We cheered and celebrated.

However, two days later we were called again as the patient had started to feel worse and was being placed on high-flow oxygen (a means to provide high amounts of oxygen without a ventilator). She was struggling to breathe. Her laboratory tests were showing very high inflammation in her system. She needed to be placed on the ventilator once again. A patient getting sick again after initial recovery can be a bad omen, and we all felt a sense of trepidation. Still, with ICU therapy, she recovered and was able to reunite with her new-born. The ICU hallways echoed for days with jubilant talk of one more countable victory that would never be forgotten.

Perhaps the words of Hippocrates come close to describing what we felt as a community: 'Wherever the art of Medicine is loved, there is love for Humanity.'

THE AFTERMATH

The COVID-19 pandemic left the city depleted on multiple fronts. Once vibrant neighbourhoods with thriving local businesses were left bereft of life as residents either stayed indoors, moved away, or had sadly passed on. A significant exodus of NYC residents to neighbouring cities or states was starkly limited to those with the means to do so. While office spaces in the towering skyscrapers of Manhattan appeared desolate in the age of remote work, at ground level, thousands of less financially advantaged families were affected by the loss of their sole breadwinners either to the economic contraction, or to COVID-19 itself. In many cases, the breadwinner was also the caretaker for the family unit, and minority women were disproportionately represented in this group (Frye, 2020). New York's unique demography meant that this problem was further magnified by another factor—a large fraction of the working class were immigrants, and hundreds of thousands of these were undocumented. Multiple food relief organizations have reported that as much as 75 percent of their clients were going hungry (Amandolare et al., 2020). The impact of this loss of income on families was unquantifiable and long-lasting.

It is notable that the loss of life related to COVID-19 is not limited to those who died from the disease and its complications. Estimates of excess deaths during the period of 11 March–2 May 2020 were around 24,000 in NYC alone, with 22% (over 5,000) of those not attributed to COVID-19. The United States suffered some 275,000 more deaths than the five-year average between 1 March and 16 August, compared to 169,000 confirmed COVID-19 deaths during that period (Giattino et al., 2021).

That said, healthcare leaders were quick to assess that while the first wave subsided in April, it was a matter of time before it was to return. Preparations continued without respite, including stockpiling ventilators and PPE, building relationships for resource-sharing and expanding telemedicine capabilities.

THE FUTURE

The NYC experience brought into the spotlight the weaknesses that are currently inherent in the US healthcare system—surge capacity, inequity in healthcare access, supply chain vulnerability, and coordination between healthcare systems, to name a few. Emerging from this disaster scenario, it would be an oversight not to recognize and continue to strengthen these vulnerabilities.

NOTE

This contributed chapter was accepted for publication in this refereed edited volume on May 9, 2021.

1   The opinions expressed are their own and do not represent the official position of their employers or the Editors.

REFERENCES

Amandolare S., L. Gallagher, J. Bowles, and E. Dvorkin, (2020), "Under Threat & Left Out: NYC's Immigrants and the Coronavirus Crisis," *Center for an Urban Future (CUF)*, https://nycfuture.org/research/under-threat-and-left-out.

Basu, A., T. Zinger, K. Inglima, K. Woo, O. Atie, L. Yurasits, B. See, and M. Aguero-Rosenfeld, (2020), "Performance of Abbott ID Now COVID-19 Rapid Nucleic Acid Amplification Test Using Nasopharyngeal Swabs Transported in Viral Transport Media and Dry Nasal Swabs in a New York City Academic Institution," *Journal of Clinical Microbiology*, 58(8), DOI: 10.1128/JCM.01136-20

Cuza B., (2020), "Why NYC Says Widespread Coronavirus Testing May Be Counter-Productive," *NY1*, https://www.ny1.com/nyc/all-boroughs/coronavirus/2020/04/06/coronavirus-testing-centers-testing-for-coronavirus-why-is-it-not-widespread-in-nyc.

Giattino, C., H. Ritchie, M. Roser, E. Ortiz-Ospina, and J. Hasell, (2021), "Excess Mortality during the Coronavirus Pandemic (COVID-19)," *Our World in Data*, https://ourworldindata.org/excess-mortality-covid.

Frye J., (2020), "On the Frontlines at Work and at Home: The Disproportionate Economic Effects of the Coronavirus Pandemic on Women of Color," *The Center for American Progress*, https://www.americanprogress.org/issues/women/reports/2020/04/23/483846/frontlines-work-home/.

New York State Department of Health, *New York State Community Health Indicator Reports (CHIRS): Annual Median Household Income in US Dollars, 2016*, https://webbi1.health.ny.gov/SASStoredProcess/guest?_program=/EBI/PHIG/apps/chir_dashboard/chir_dashboard&p=it&ind_id=Ng100.

NYC Health, 2021, *Summary of Current New York City COVID-19 Guidance for Isolation, Quarantine and Transmission-Based Precautions*, https://www1.nyc.gov/assets/doh/downloads/pdf/imm/covid-19-provider-quarantine-precautions.pdf.

O'Donnell M., (2006), "In Queens, It's the Glorious 4th, and 6th, and 16th, and 25th…," *The New York Times*, https://www.nytimes.com/2006/07/04/nyregion/04fourth.html.

Port Authority NYNJ, *Data & Statistics*, 2021, https://www.panynj.gov/airports/en/statistics-general-info.html.

U.S. Census Bureau, Quick Facts, (2021), New York city, New York, https://www.census.gov/quickfacts/newyorkcitynewyork.

Web.mta.info, (2021), mta.info | Facts and Figures, http://web.mta.info/nyct/facts/ffsubway.htm.

Weber A., (2013), "Queens," NewYork.com, https://web.archive.org/web/20150513065643/http://www.newyork.com/articles/neighborhoods/queens-72876/.

Willman D., (2020), "Contamination at CDC Lab Delayed Rollout of Coronavirus Tests," *The Washington Post*, https://www.washingtonpost.com/investigations/contamination-at-cdc-lab-delayed-rollout-of-coronavirus-tests/2020/04/18/fd7d3824-7139-11ea-aa80-c2470c6b2034_story.html.

10

COVID-19 HERD IMMUNITY AND ROLE OF VACCINES

Arnab Ghosh, Kapil Goyal,
and Mini P. Singh

CONCEPT OF HERD IMMUNITY

Herd immunity is a key determinant for measuring resistance against transmission of an infectious agent within a given population. Optimum levels of herd immunity to halt an epidemic or pandemic is reached when the proportion of immune individuals is sufficiently high so that the susceptible fraction of population does not contract the disease as transmission is blocked at the immune population level (Desai and Majumder, 2013). The concept of herd immunity has been schematically presented in Figure 10.1. The herd immunity threshold is determined by the parameter, the "basic reproduction number" or R_0 and is mathematically expressed as $(1 - 1/R_0)$. R_0 is defined as the average expected number of secondary cases infected from a single index case introduced into a totally susceptible population. Considering this definition, an R_0 value of greater than 1 implies that each index case attributes to more than 1 secondary case and the transmission is high. An R_0 value of less than 1 denotes a declining trend of transmission as each index case transmits the infection to less than 1 secondary case. However, the reproduction number for an agent does not remain constant. As the epidemic or pandemic continues, a part of the population may become partially immunized, even in the absence of an effective vaccine, due to natural infection and the average number of secondary infections from a single infective index case decrease. Such changes in transmission

DOI: 10.4324/9781003218807-12

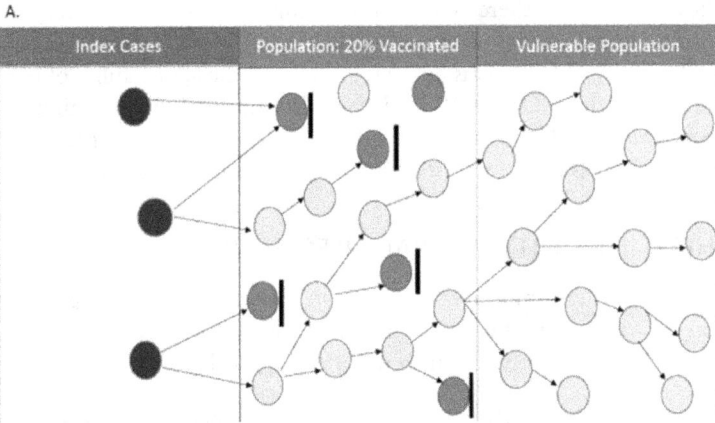

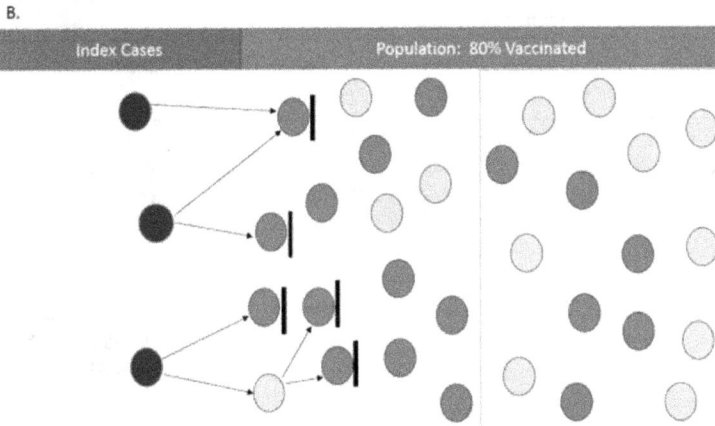

Fig 1. Schematic Representation of spread of infection with R_0 of 2 in
A. Population immunity at 20%
B. Population immunity at 80%

Codes: ● : Index Case ● : Vaccinated ○ :Susceptible ▌ : Transmission blockade

Figure 10.1 Schematic representation of spread of infection with R_0 of 2 in. A)
Population immunity with 20%. (B) Population immunity with 80%

dynamics of infection are represented by the term "Effective reproduction number or R_e" (Delamater et al., 2019).

To have clarity over the concept of herd immunity in a novel viral infection like Severe Acute Respiratory Syndrome Coronavirus-2

(SARS-CoV-2), there is a need to examine the herd immunity for extensively studied viral infections, like measles, polio, small pox, and influenza A/H1N1. This helps us understand the applicability of herd immunity in COVID-19 and the differences in herd immunity between COVID-19 and viral infections where the role of the herd immunity has been well established for eradication or elimination.

HERD IMMUNITY IN VIRAL INFECTIONS

Metrics of herd immunity differ between viral infections depending on the virus properties, the immunity induced, and the vaccine efficacy. The basic reproduction number (R_0) and the calculated herd

Table 10.1 Comparison of herd immunity threshold of viruses with pandemic or epidemic potential

Virus	Basic reproduction no (R0)	Mean herd immunity threshold	Current status
Measles	12–18	93%	Eliminated in many developed countries with sporadic outbreaks; Regular outbreaks in developing countries
Polio	5–7	83%	Eradicated
Small Pox	5–7	83%	Eradicated
Influenza A/ H1N1 (2009)	1.4–1.5	30%	Intermittent outbreaks
Ebola (2015)	1.5–2.5	50%	Limited to outbreaks in Africa at present
SARS (2003)	2–2.75	60%	End of the epidemic in 2004
MERS	01	Unknown	2566 cases till Dec 2020 – most cases from Saudi Arabia
SARS-CoV-2	2–4	70%	Current ongoing pandemic

immunity threshold of viral infections with pandemic or epidemic potentials have been summarized in Table 10.1. Of the listed viruses, the measles virus has the highest R_0 and requires more than 90% of the population to be immune in the community for its elimination, preferably in the form of vaccination. However, it should be noted that natural infection with measles induces lifelong immunity in contrast to a SARS-CoV-2 infection. Besides, the measles vaccine, after a standard 2-dose regimen, has an excellent efficacy of approximately 95%, with long-lasting immunity. Thus, the immune response, both antibody and cell mediated, to measles infection and vaccination is robust. Sporadic breakthrough outbreaks in communities, after measles elimination, has been the result of suboptimal vaccine coverage in subpopulations and introduction of susceptible population into the community (Dimala et al., 2019). Moreover, asymptomatic cases of measles in a susceptible population are extremely rare, which implies silent transmission does not occur in measles. This results in accurate R_0 calculation and herd immunity threshold prediction for measles. Similarly, if we consider small pox with a crude fatality rate of 30% caused by variola, a double-stranded DNA virus, eradication was possible because of an effective vaccine, a stable virus genome, and transmission occurring primarily from symptomatic patients which made containment and surveillance successful, quite unlike the SARS-CoV-2 virus (Metzger et al., 2015).

The case of poliomyelitis eradication is a completely different scenario as polio can cause asymptomatic infections which can transmit the disease, and the injectable polio vaccine does not inhibit transmission. Eradication of poliomyelitis has been achieved by inducing herd immunity by indirect vaccination. In this case, indirect vaccination refers to the oral polio vaccine (OPV) given in mass vaccination campaigns and the OPV strain being transmitted feco-orally to non-vaccinated contacts of vaccinees inducing mucosal immunity. The IgA-mediated mucosal immunity in the gut protects against infection by wild polio virus even in non-vaccinated ones, which the injectable inactivated polio vaccine cannot induce (Kew et al., 2018). The circulation of the vaccine virus in the community, in the environment, and from vaccinated to non-vaccinated individuals amplifies the proportion of immune population achieving herd immunity.

Considering the influenza, A/H1N1, there is an availability of an effective treatment in the form of oseltamivir, a neuraminidase inhibitor which not only lessens disease severity but also decreases transmission by inhibiting viral replication. The inactivated quadrivalent vaccine covers all the circulating influenza virus strains. The strategy is to vaccinate annually by updating the vaccine strains, depending on the changes in the circulating wild strains, due to antigenic drift. This maintains an optimum level of immunity in the vaccinated population, even if there is antigenic variation between influenza strains (Houser et al., 2015). Thus COVID-19 herd immunity presents to us a totally different scenario compared to the viruses which have already been eradicated or are on the verge of elimination.

COVID-19 HERD IMMUNITY: HOW IS IT DIFFERENT?

When the SARS-CoV-2 outbreak started in the Wuhan district of China, at the end of December 2019, there had been close to 170 million confirmed cases worldwide till May 2021, with more than 3.5 million deaths. India, which is currently in the declining phase of the second wave of the pandemic, has recorded more than 27 million cases with more than 0.3 million deaths till May 2021. The question now is how close countries like India, Brazil, and the United States are (which constitutes almost 60% of the total COVID-19 burden worldwide) in achieving herd immunity (WHO, 2021a). With almost 17 vaccines cleared by regulatory agencies in at least 1 country for full usage, and several vaccine candidates in different phases of trial, there is a need to know what proportion of population in a country needs to be vaccinated to break the chain of transmission and prevent subsequent resurgences.

COMPLEXITY IN CALCULATING COVID-19 HERD IMMUNITY THRESHOLD

Although R_0 is a simple and valuable concept in determining the herd immunity threshold, the actual scenario for SARS-CoV-2 is complex. First, the numerical value of R_0 has shown variations among countries, and also subpopulations attributed to factors like population density, population structure, compliance to COVID-19-appropriate behaviour, and lock-down impositions which could directly affect SARS-CoV-2 transmission. There are wide variations in R_0 of SARS-CoV-2: WHO estimates of

SARS-CoV-2 R_0 in Wuhan during the early part of pandemic ranged from 1.4 to 2.5, while median R_0 value was initially 5.8 in the United States and ranged between 3.6 and 6.1 in some European nations (Rahman et al., 2020; Ke et al., 2021). Thus, a single absolute value of R_0 in determining the immune threshold for a widely diverse country like India will also be incorrect.

However, with the introduction of vaccination and occurrence of two waves of the pandemic in most countries, the numerical value of reproduction number is bound to change as R_0, by definition, is calculated in a totally susceptible population. In addition, the degree of exposure of diverse population subgroups to SARS-CoV-2 is also different; for example, the young adult age groups are more prone to be exposed to the virus as compared to the elderly and the paediatric population. This will lead to variations in the calculation of the resulting immune status, due to natural infection in various strata of the population. Moreover, the interaction or contact rates among individuals, among different sections of the society, depending on the social strata, also differ. So, calculation of reproduction number based on a simplistic calculation may not be a true representation of the community protection. Reproduction number in the initial part of the first wave of the pandemic was close to 3 in most countries which dropped down to a range of 1.38–1.45 by three months due to lockdown measures and rising proportion of immune population. At present, during the ongoing second wave of the pandemic in India, the current reproduction number in all states stands at approximately 1.3 with values of more than 1.5 in some states (Ranjan et al., 2021). Moreover, testing for SARS-CoV-2 by real-time reverse transcriptase PCR is not uniform throughout, and actual number of cases may be greater than the reported number, particularly in rural areas. This means the numbers are representative of an optimistic scenario as true rates of transmission may be much higher.

One of the major hindrances in calculating the reproduction number and determining the actual rate of SARS-CoV-2 transmission is the relatively high proportion of asymptomatic cases of COVID-19 infection. Approximately 40–45% of SARS-CoV-2 cases can be asymptomatic, and asymptomatic cases can efficiently transmit infection to susceptible individuals (Kaneko et al., 2020; Great Barrington Declaration, 2021). Asymptomatic cases are more prone to spread the infection as they remain undetected and have higher contact rates. The inclusion of asymptomatic cases in studying the transmission dynamics is difficult in the absence of uniform screening of the entire population, and the calculated reproduction number is based on data comprising mostly of symptomatic cases. One of the effective strategies of downregulating transmission is screening a large number of the population so that the asymptomatic cases are detected early and isolated. However, it is worth mentioning that more asymptomatic cases in a given community implies that the population will probably attain herd immunity threshold earlier than expected due to higher proportion of immune population.

NATURE OF COVID-19 IMMUNE RESPONSE AFFECTING HERD IMMUNITY

SARS-CoV-2 infection and vaccination induces antibody responses to viral proteins. The antibodies against the spike protein receptor-binding domain (RBD) elicit virus neutralizing response and are presumably correlates of protection against further SARS-CoV-2 infections. However, it has been observed that these anti-SARS-CoV-2 antibodies start to decline within 3 months of infection, particularly in milder cases. So, the humoral immune responses after SARS-CoV-2 are not a long-lasting protective immunity. In fact, reinfection by SARS-CoV-2 has been reported 5–6 months after the first episode (Kellam and Barclay, 2020). The duration of the neutralizing antibody response in response to vaccination is under evaluation as it has been barely 6 months since vaccination has started. Studies regarding duration of antibody response in SARS-CoV-2 vaccination will be able to bridge the gap in knowledge in the future. Once the time interval during which the neutralizing antibody response decays to suboptimum levels is known, it will help in defining the timing of booster dosage for a given vaccine. There is a need to look into the cell-mediated arm of adaptive immunity against SARS-CoV-2 which is equally important as the humoral arm in controlling a viral infection.

SARS-COV-2 VACCINATION: ROLE IN HERD IMMUNITY

The only feasible way of achieving herd immunity for an infection is through large-scale immunization. Inducing immunity by natural infection and gradually gaining herd immunity threshold has been suggested in the Great Barrington Declaration by three scientists, Martin Kuldorff, Sunetra Gupta, and Jay Bhattacharya (Great Barrington Declaration, 2021). The declaration is based on focused protection of the vulnerable population, like the elderly and those with comorbidities, and allowing the young healthy population to resume normal life to minimize the collateral damage caused by complete lockdown measures. By this declaration, the young healthy adult population is expected to become immune by natural infection, and once this group, which comprises a greater part of the population, gains herd immunity, it prevents infection transmission to the vulnerable community. However, the concept is flawed in many aspects.

COVID-19 complications, including mortality, are mediated by the cytokines activating the inflammatory cascade, which cannot be predicted accurately beforehand. Young adults too can have severe disease effects, even resulting in death, as have been observed during the second wave of the pandemic. So, in a highly populated country like India, encouraging exposure in any subgroup of population will definitely increase mortality in both vulnerable and non-vulnerable groups. In addition, natural infection due to SARS-CoV-2 is associated with loss of germinal centres in spleen and lymph nodes which implies natural immunity due to COVID-19 may not be long-lasting. This phenomenon is caused by the systemic inflammatory response accompanying infection and is not expected post-vaccination (Kaneko et al., 2020). So, achieving herd immunity without increase in COVID-19 mortality and morbidity will require implementation of a widely adopted vaccination policy.

The SARS-CoV-2 vaccines approved for full usage in multiple countries after clearing the three phases of trial have been listed in Table 10.2. Considering vaccine efficacy for preventing COVID-19 infection, all these vaccines have at least 70% efficacy. The two vaccines that have been extensively used in India, COVISHIELD (Serum Institute of India) and COVAXIN (Bharat-Biotech), have shown efficacy of 70% and 78% in preventing disease, respectively, and an acceptable safety profile (Ella et al., 2021; New Indian Express, 2021). Subsequent studies should focus on the durability of the vaccine-induced immune response so as to decide on the schedule of a booster dose, if at all required.

Table 10.2 SARS-CoV-2 vaccines approved for full usage in multiple countries (at least 5)

Name of vaccines	Mechanism of action	Manufacturer	Country of origin	Phase III trial efficacy (%)
Comirnaty (BNT162b2)	mRNA encoding Spike protein	Pfizer, BioNTech, Fosun Pharma	Multinational	95
Moderna COVID-19 vaccine (mRNA-1273)	mRNA encoding Spike protein	Moderna, NIAID	United States	94
COVID-19 Astrazeneca Vaccine	Adenovirus vector encoding spike protein	Oxford/ Astrazeneca (Vaxzevria) Serum Institute India (Covishield)	United Kingdom	80
SputnikV	Adenovirus vector encoding spike protein	Gamaleya Research Institute, Acellena Contract Drug Research and Development	Russia	91.6
Covaxin	Inactivated vaccine	Bharat Biotech	India	81
CoronaVac	Inactivated vaccine	Sinovac	China	50.6
BBIBP-CorV	Inactivated vaccine	Sinopharm (Beijing)	China	78.1
Janssen Vaccine	Adenovirus vector vaccine (single dose)	Johnson & Johnson	Netherlands, Belgium	66
CanSino COVID-19 Vaccine	Adenovirus vectored vaccine	CanSino Biologics	China	68.8

Considering a mean vaccine efficacy (V_e) of 75%, and a current reproduction number of approximately 1.5, the percentage of population that needs to be vaccinated will be 44% based on the formula $(1 - 1/R)/V_e$. India with a huge population of 136 crores (1.36 billion) will thus require approximately 120 crore (1.2 billion) vaccine doses for a standard 2-dose regimen. India started vaccination from January 2021 with a targeted approach for health-care workers, frontline workers, and persons with comorbidities and old age; by March 2021 about 96 lakh (or 9.6 million) people received 2 doses of vaccine, but that constituted only 0.7% of the total population (WHO, 2021b). A low vaccine coverage has been one of the contributory factors behind the high burden of cases during the second wave of the pandemic. Till the end of May 2021 India has fully vaccinated 42 million people or 3.1% of the population. To reach the optimum herd immunity threshold, upscaling vaccine production will be of utmost importance. India has started vaccinating all above 18 years of age, thus also increasing the demand for vaccines. Vaccinating all people above 18 years will cover 60% of the population and may be the cornerstone for preventing COVID-19 surges in the near future. The unimmunized pockets of population and the paediatric age group can be vaccinated subsequently after the safety and immunogenicity profile in children have been established.

IDEAL VACCINE FOR HERD IMMUNITY

An ideal vaccine to achieve herd immunity threshold for SARS-CoV-2 would be able to prevent transmission of the virus from vaccinated individuals. The vaccines currently approved for full usage are given intramuscularly. They are either a viral vectored vaccine carrying the spike glycoprotein or mRNA encoding spike glycoprotein or inactivated vaccines which are not proven to induce mucosal immunity and block viral transmission. In this scenario, a live attenuated vaccine given intranasally will be able to induce IgA-mediated mucosal immunity as well as mucosal cell-mediated T-cell immune responses preventing infection and transmission as seen with OPV. Such a vaccine will be non-invasive and needle-free and will be an ideal vaccine for the paediatric population. The two intranasal vaccine candidates BBV-154 and CoviVac which are live attenuated chimpanzee adenovirus carrying SARS-CoV-2 spike (S) protein gene are in Phase I trial in India and the United Kingdom, respectively.

SARS-COV-2 VARIANT EFFECTS ON HERD IMMUNITY

Into 1.5 years of the pandemic, the SARS-CoV-2 virus has shown to undergo mutations in different parts of the genome like spike, envelope, nucleoprotein, and replicase genes. The most significant of these mutations are those in the RBD of the spike glycoprotein, the binding site for neutralizing antibody generated post infection as well as post vaccination. Mutations in the RBD decrease the neutralizing antibody affinity to these binding sites which helps the virus in immune evasion and increase transmissibility, and the variants are termed as "variants of concern (VOCs)". One of the most prevalent VOCs is the UK variant or B.1.1.7 (Alpha Variant) lineage carrying signature mutations and deletion in and around the spike protein (N501Y, P681H and 59/60 del), in addition to several others in different parts of the genome. It has now been reported from more than 100 countries including India. Other important VOCs include the South Africa variant or B.1.353 (Beta Variant) lineage, the Brazilian variant or P.1 lineage, and the double variant originating in India or B.1.617 (Delta Variant) with additional mutations in the immunodominant regions of spike protein. It has been observed that convalescent sera from recovered patients of the COVID-19 Wuhan strain and sera from vaccinated people have decreased neutralizing activity against B.1.1.7 and B.1.253 (Harvey et al., 2021). More than 50% of cases of reinfection have been caused by variant strains worldwide. The double mutant has been detected in re-infected patients and in vaccinated individuals with breakthrough infections in India. Since the variant strains pose a major threat to herd immunity, genomic surveillance of SARS-CoV-2 by whole genome sequencing will be a key strategy for detecting the emergence of these variants and bring modifications in vaccine design in future if the neutralizing capacity of the current vaccine to variant strains drop to suboptimum levels. Genomic surveillance will also help to detect emergence of variants that may arise due to vaccine-induced antibody pressure. However, vaccination on a mass scale is the most effective way to prevent the emergence of variants as vaccine-induced herd immunity will cause reduction of circulation of SARS-CoV-2 strains and minimize transmission, leading to lower viral replication in the community and thus lower rates of mutations.

To summarize, although achieving herd immunity threshold calculated on the basis of reproduction number appears to be a promising concept, the actual scenario is much more complex than expected. As mentioned previously, with an efficacy of 75% for the Indian vaccines, at least 45% of the population is required to have herd immunity considering a reproduction number of 1.5. But only 50% population being infected and/or vaccinated will not ensure the end of the COVID-19 pandemic, the reasons being waning immunity in COVID-19 infection or immunization, emergence of immune evading variants, and uneven roll-out of vaccines. So only focusing on herd immunity may not provide a solution in ending this pandemic.

As the second wave of the pandemic is nearing an end in India, an extensive sero-surveillance to detect IgG antibodies against SARS-CoV-2 is needed to be carried out, covering all strata of the population, for example, urban slums, urban non–slums, and rural areas. As there are regions with comparatively lower number of real-time PCR tests, the actual burden of cases is unknown, and the sero-survey will provide indirect evidence regarding this aspect. In addition, it will help to highlight the immunologically naïve population; mass-scale vaccination strategy should be targeted to this group. With vaccines being targeted at adults only at present, the paediatric population will still remain susceptible and act as a conduit for transmission causing further resurgences. Sero-surveillance should thus also include the paediatric age group, to detect the baseline sero-prevalence in children. Vaccine trial for children has started, and vaccination will be implemented between 2 and 18 years of age depending on the safety and efficacy of the trial.

One of the major hurdles in achieving large-scale vaccine coverage is the vaccine hesitancy among common people. Since COVID-19 vaccine development has occurred at an unprecedented pace as compared to other infections where vaccine development had taken years to decades, people are still not totally convinced regarding the safety and efficacy of the approved vaccines. People should be convinced that among vaccinated individuals, rates of mortality, ICU admission, and hospitalization are lower as compared to non-vaccinated individuals (Haas et al., 2021). Safety profile of different vaccines are gradually becoming more evident. Bringing the scientific information into the public domain in simple layman's language will be able to alleviate the doubts in people's minds. Ensuring uninterrupted supply and availability of the two doses for all will also help in overcoming vaccine hesitancy.

Even if the predicted herd immunity figures are achieved, the SARS-CoV-2 virus is not going to be easily eradicated or eliminated, in the near future. Moreover, SARS-CoV-2 has animal reservoirs and have already caused outbreaks in mink farms in Europe. This raises the possibility of establishment of mammalian transmission and spillover to the human population. This means veterinary surveillance may become an important strategy in our efforts of elimination.

The best of efforts will enable preventing major outbreaks and will include continuous testing for SARS-CoV-2 on a large-scale basis by real-time PCR, even when transmission is low, tracking and isolating positive patients, maintaining proper masking practices and social distancing strategy, along with vaccination through an even and uninterrupted distribution. The COVID-19-appropriate behaviours need to be reinforced in public regularly as complacency sets in in vaccinated individuals. The strategy for booster doses for different vaccines should be worked out, particularly for the vulnerable population, considering there can be vaccine shortage due to rising demand. Till a level of herd immunity strong enough to prevent resurgences is achieved, focus should be directed to reduce disease severity and transmission blockade by control measures and will require a combined strong-willed effort from the scientific community as well as from all strata of the general population.

NOTE

This contributed chapter was accepted for publication in this refereed edited volume on July 1, 2021.

REFERENCES

Delamater, P.L., E.J. Street, T.F. Leslie, Y. Yang, and K.H. Jacobsen, (2019), "Complexity of the basic reproduction number (R_0)," *Emerg Infect Dis*, 25(1), pp. 1–4.

Desai, A.N., and M.S. Majumder, (2013), "What is herd immunity?" *JAMA*, 324(20), p. 2113.

Dimala, C.A., B.M. Kadia, M.A.M. Nji, and N.N. Bechem, (2021), "Factors associated with measles resurgence in the United States in the post-elimination era," *Sci Rep* 11, p. 51.

Ella, R, S. Reddy, H. Jogdand, V. Sarangi, B. Ganneru, and S. Prasad, et al., (2021), "Safety and immunogenicity of an inactivated SARS-CoV-2 vaccine, BBV152: interim results from a double-blind, randomised, multicentre, phase 2 trial, and 3-month follow-up of a double-blind, randomised phase 1 trial," *Lancet Infect* Dis 21, pp. 950–961.

Great Barrington Declaration, (2021), https://gbdeclaration.org/. (Accessed on May 10 2021).

Haas, E.J., F.J. Angulo, J.M. McLaughlin, Anis E, Singer SR, Khan F, et al. (2021), "Impact and effectiveness of mRNA BNT162b2 vaccine against SARS-CoV-2 infections and COVID-19 cases, hospitalisations, and deaths following a nationwide vaccination campaign in Israel: an observational study using national surveillance data," *Lancet*, 397(10287), pp. 1819–1829.

Harvey, W.T., A.M. Carabelli, B. Jackson, R.K. Gupta, E.C. Thomson, E.M. Harrison, C. Ludden, R. Reeve, and A. Rambaut, (2021), "COVID-19 genomics UK (COG-UK) Consortium, Peacock SJ, Robertson DL. SARS-CoV-2 variants, spike mutations and immune escape," *Nat Rev Microbiol*, 19(7), pp. 409–424.

Houser, K., Subbarao, K., (2015), Influenza vaccines: challenges and solutions. *Cell Host Microbe*, 17(3), pp. 295–300.

Kaneko, N., H.H. Kuo, J. Boucau, J.R. Farmer, H. Allard-Chamard, and V.S. Mahajan, et al., (2020), "Loss of Bcl-6-Expressing T Follicular helper cells and germinal centers in COVID-19," Cell, Oct 1, 183(1), pp. 143–157.e13.

Ke, R., E. Romero-Severson, S. Sanche and N. Hengartne, (2021), "Estimating the reproductive number R_0 of SARS-CoV-2 in the United States and eight European countries and implications for vaccination," *J Theor Biol*, 517, p. 110621.

Kellam, P., and W. Barclay, (2020), "The dynamics of humoral immune responses following SARS-CoV-2 infection and the potential for reinfection," *J Gen Virol*, Aug, 101(8), pp. 791–797.

Kew, O., and M. Pallansch, (2018), "Breaking the last chains of poliovirus transmission: progress and challenges in global polio eradication," *Annu Rev Virol*, 5(1), pp. 427–451.

Metzger W.G., C. Köhler, B. Mordmüller, (2015), "Lessons from a modern review of the smallpox eradication files," *J R Soc Med*, 108(12), pp. 473–477.

Rahman, B., E. Sadraddin and A. Porreca, (2020), "The basic reproduction number of SARS-CoV-2 in Wuhan is about to die out, how about the rest of the World?" *Rev Med Virol*, 30(4), p. e2111.

Ranjan, R., A. Sharma, and M.K. Verma, (2021), "Characterization of the second wave of COVID-19 in India," medRxiv 2021.04.17.21255665, https://doi.org/10.1101/2021.04.17.21255665.

The New Indian Express, (2020), "Oxford vaccine Covishield shows 70% efficacy against Covid-19," https://www.newindianexpress.com/world/2020/nov/23/oxford-vaccine-covishield-shows-70-efficacy-against-covid-19-2226993.html.

WHO, (2021a), "WHO coronavirus (COVID-19) dashboard," https://covid19.who.int/.

WHO, (2021b), "COVID-19 vaccine tracker and landscape," https://www.who.int/publications/m/item/draft-landscape-of-covid-19-candidate-vaccines.

VIRTUAL FIRESIDE CONVERSATIONS WITH PROFESSIONALS AND BUSINESS LEADERS

With Co-Editors Aurobindo Ghosh (AG), Amit Haldar (AH), and Kalyan Bhaumik (KB)

Conversation with **Dr Sushmita Roy Chowdhury (SRC), Head, Pulmonary Department, Fortis Hospital, Kolkata, India**

1. AH: Do prophylactic medications have any role in COVID?

SRC: The basic principle of prevention better than cure forms the basis of looking for prophylactic treatment in any disease. Search for prophylactic agents started early in the case of the highly infective COVID-19. HCQ (hydroxychloroquine) was the first agent that garnered a lot of interest, especially in India. Its easy availability, known safety profile, and affordability were the key reasons. The rationale for its use was derived from results of 100 Chinese patients with COVID-19 where the group that received chloroquine had reduction in exacerbation of pneumonia, delayed viral clearing, and symptoms (Colson et al., 2020). China was the first country to include chloroquine in prophylaxis. Based on this premise, hydroxychloroquine should also work in the same way with a better safety profile, lower cost, and favourable preclinical data. HCQ was adopted as a medicine for prophylaxis by the ICMR. However, due to flaws in methodology of clinical trials, incorrect dosing, improper duration, and frequency of administration, HCQ failed to

DOI: 10.4324/9781003218807-13

demonstrate appreciable benefits in preventing infection and was dropped from national guidelines of India. Similarly, ivermectin, a safe antihelminthic (helminth means worms) drug used in treatment of strongyloidiasis was found by Caly et al. (2020) to have in vitro activity against SARS CoV2 followed by a pilot clinical trial by Chaccour et al. (2021) that showed a tendency to reduce viral load and early recovery from hyposmia in the group treated with a single dose of 400mcg/kg of ivermectin. Current evidence does not lend any rationale for continuing these agents for prophylaxis, and these have been removed from revised national guidelines in India.

2. AH: What is the main issue with remdesivir?

SRC: Remdesivir, a repurposed drug, was initially used for treatment of hepatitis C and Ebola. When the pandemic struck, remdesivir was used as an investigational drug against COVID. It was widely used until the interim report from the WHO Solidarity trial showed no mortality benefit from it in hospitalized patients. Interestingly, the ACTT-1 trial in the United States and Recovery trial in the United Kingdom reported shortened time to recovery with remdesivir previously (Beigel et al., 2020).

Our own clinical observation has been the same in both the first and second waves. This is even more evident if it is given early in the viral phase within the first 7 days. Not only do most patients have early defervescence, they also have better sense of well-being.

I feel the Solidarity trial needs to be re-evaluated with respect to how many people on remdesivir received it within the first 7 days of illness and their rates of recovery.

3. AH: What is the role of steroids in treatment of COVID-19?

SRC: Steroids have certainly been the cornerstone of effective and affordable treatment in the pandemic. Its easy over-the-counter availability made it the most misused drug too. The best period of its use is in the second week in patients with moderate to severe pulmonary involvement presenting with hypoxia. Those who are prescribed steroids too early, or self-medicated with it in order to relieve symptoms of fever and myalgia invariably worsened. Also, at the height of the pandemic, when hospital beds were scarce, many general physicians commenced steroids at home. Sometimes the patients continued it beyond the prescribed period due to the sense of well-being and its easy availability.

4. AH: How did you do triage and manage the COVID patients in an ICU set-up?

SRC: Intensive care treatment for COVID pneumonia is reserved for those having severe pneumonia with respiratory failure (Type I at presentation). Most of these patients have happy hypoxia (nil or minimal symptoms) or clinical distress despite severe hypoxia. The aim of oxygenation is to keep saturations above 92% with lowest amount of oxygen. Up to 10/minute requirement of oxygen with no respiratory distress is well managed with face masks and non-rebreathing masks. This is done in addition to awake proning (a posture of lying flat with face downwards) of patients. Higher oxygen requirements are enabled with HFNO (High-flow Nasal Oxygen) which not only helps in providing higher concentration of oxygen (via a nasal device), it also helps to prevent claustrophobia associated with face masks and enables the patient to eat and drink with the oxygen supply in place. It is well tolerated at higher flow rates too, but we have observed a slightly increased rate of spontaneous pneumomediastinum (air in the middle of chest between the lungs and around the heart) in the second wave in such patients. Non-invasive ventilation is helpful in patients with increased work of breathing, in moderate ARDS (Acute Respiratory Distress Syndrome), those with associated COPD (Chronic Obstructive Pulmonary Disease) and Type 2 Respiratory failure, OSA (Obstructive Sleep Apnea)with OHS, and heart failure patients. Alternating between HFNO and NIV (Non-invasive Ventilation) seems the best tolerated option in many patients. Mechanical ventilation has been a challenging modality. We found that early elective intubation outcomes are better than delayed intubation in those who remained in severe ARDS with P/F ratio below 100 and increased work of breathing despite being on NIV or those who are drowsy at presentation with severe ARDS.

Only a small subset of these patients, who fail despite a good trial of 48–72 hours of prone mechanical ventilation, are considered as candidates for ECMO (Extracorporeal Membrane Oxygenation, a life support machine). Successful weaning from ECMO on an average takes 18–19 days. (personal experience). Age is never a barrier to choosing modality of treatment in our set-up. However, in those with advanced comorbidities such as malignancy, ILD (Interstitial Lung Disease), and severe COPD, the decision to mechanically ventilate is taken after prior discussion and ceiling of care established at NIV in most patients.

5. AH: What is mucormycosis?

SRC: Mucor is an opportunistic fungus which usually infects severely debilitated, diabetic, and immunosuppressed individuals. The infection most commonly starts in the paranasal sinuses. This is likely due to poor drainage of this area. The fungus causes angioinvasion and spreads rapidly to involve the maxillary bones, orbits, brain, and sometimes via the haematogenous route can affect the lungs, kidneys, and other organs. The fatality rate is very high.

6. AH: Following the COVID-19 pandemic, in India the disease has become another important health emergency. The Indian Government reported that more than 11,700 people were receiving care for mucormycosis ("black fungus") as of 25 May 2021. (Reference, Wikipedia) Why is this mucormycosis following COVID-19 India specific?

SRC: There is some complex mechanism that has led to this surge of mucormycosis. Poor host response, abundance of mucor in certain humid (Indian weather) environments, possibly poorly maintained oxygen systems transporting the fungus to nasal passages, complex siderophore opportunities provided by COVID to merrily angio invade and cause stealthy devastation are all possible. The steroids alone are not the only culprits. Strict blood sugar control and high index of suspicion in high-risk patients who complain of nasal discharge and facial numbness must call for early CT and nasal endoscopy for sampling and fungal culture.

7. AH: Does the so-called "infodemic" play a role in the pandemic development?

Infodemic creates mass hysteria. Easy accessibility to unscientific and multiple sources of information created more panic about the disease than is desirable. This led to hoarding of medicines as expensive as remdesivir and tocilizumab, equipment like oxygen cylinders and concentrators, and commencing steroids inappropriately in home settings early in the disease. This made the treatment even more difficult for the trained physicians.

I always convinced my patients with available, credible information, allaying their anxiety and by being available for online consults when they were convalescing at home. Hand-holding virtually helped immensely in reassuring and ensuring compliance to home isolation rules.

NOTE

This contributed chapter was accepted for publication in this refereed edited volume on July 1, 2021.

REFERENCES

Beigel, J., Tomashek, K., Dodd, L. E., et al., (2020), "Remdesivir for the treatment of covid-19—final report." *N Engl J Med* 2020, Oct 8. doi:10.1056/NEJMoa2007764. https://en.wikipedia.org/wiki/Mucormycosis.

Caly, L., Druce, J. D., Catton, M. G., Jans, D. A., and Wagstaff, K. M. (2020), "The FDA-approved drug ivermectin inhibits the replication of SARS-CoV-2 *in vitro*." *Antiviral Res*, 178, 104787: https://doi.org/10.1016/j.antiviral.2020.104787.Chaccour C. et al., (2021), "The effect of early treatment with ivermectin on viral load, symptoms and humoral response in patients with non-severe COVID-19: a pilot, double-blind, placebo-controlled, randomized clinical trial." *EClinicalMedicine*, 32, 100720. doi:https://doi.org/10.1016/j.eclinm.2020.100720.

Colson, P., Rolain, J.-M., and Raoult, D., (2020), "Chloroquine for the 2019 novel coronavirus SARS-CoV-2." *Int J Antimicrob Agents*, 55, 105923. doi:10.1016/j.ijantimicag.2020.105923.

VIRTUAL FIRESIDE CONVERSATIONS WITH BUSINESS LEADERS

With Co-Editors Aurobindo Ghosh (AG), Amit Haldar (AH), and Kalyan Bhaumik (KB)

Conversation with **Dr Amit Haldar (AH) on a Medical Lab: Dr Somnath Chatterjee (SC), Founder and Co-Owner, Suraksha Labs, Kolkata, India**

Suraksha, established in 1992, was one of the first diagnostics to serve all investigations under one roof. Today, it has more than 50 centres spread across many states and houses one of the largest referral labs in the country. Equipped with a state-of-the-art molecular lab, it has conducted more than 250,000 RT-PCR Tests for COVID-19.

1. AH: What are the factors that you took into account when the first outbreak started? Did you think of multiple waves and prepare? With the second wave of COVID-19, how did you expand capacity temporarily and keep the staff motivated?

SC: Factors that we took into account were as follows:

1. Learnt and deployed new technologies in the Molecular Lab.
2. Expanded the team and created protocols.

DOI: 10.4324/9781003218807-14

3. Started working 24×7 in shifts.
4. Ensured sufficient supply of consumables.
5. Prepared logistical needs.

Honestly speaking, the pressure of the work was so much that we hardly had time to think about a second wave. Extremely anxious patients and their families were waiting for reports that we had to deliver. It was a Herculean task.

In the lab, when COVID-related workload had just started to normalize, the second wave descended upon us with surprising abruptness.

The only way of motivating our staff was to stand with them. Our CEO and I were the most frequent visitors to that floor. Additionally, our CEO led the process from the front and got the entire workflow automated. Starting from a Phlebotomist to the Microbiologist, all had joined forces to fight alike, the Suraksha team of "COVID" Warriors. We also introduced performance-based financial incentives.

2. AH: One important aspect of COVID-19 has been the time it takes to do the RT-PCR test; how do you prioritize if there are huge number of tests coming?

SC: Well, it does. The two steps—Extraction and PCR—take around two hours despite major automation done during both. They run in batches of 96, so it takes significant time to prepare and then run it. However, there were always critical cases where we have produced a report within 6 hours, an impossibly short Turnaround Time (TAT). Over time, we have managed to completely automate the process. So, handling a fair volume is not a challenge anymore. When there are emergency samples, we run a process to fast-track the samples. We have two entirely separate runs earmarked in the day to facilitate the emergency samples with the logistics team always kept in the loop. Separate WhatsApp groups have been created to keep track of the same, where Microbiologists are always involved. We also built a chain of command as to who could request an emergency report. A COVID helpline was set up and also a number of WhatsApp channels for patients to reach us.

3. AH: How do you assure consistency of the test results even though changing directives might be coming in from the medical advisory board or government?

SC: To begin with one validates both the extraction kit and the PCR along with their consumables, followed by dry runs before going live. The samples are checked by both the ICMR and State government. Concordance is notified. We use an external Quality Control (QC) and do interlab tests at regular intervals. Directives have never been about the technology within the lab, which remained clear from the beginning. There is an SOP for everything. Highly qualified scientists work on it. However, directives have come for pricing, billing software, portal uploading etc. So, they are standard changes that one goes through as they scale up.

4. AH: How do you keep yourself abreast of new research and new tests coming up in this rapidly changing medical research world?

SC: This is the only enjoyable part of this experience. Since the entire medical world was focussed to find a solution, astounding work was done to quickly introduce the test kits for doing the RT-PCR. Virtual seminars, both national and international, helped in a long way. Leading scientists were explaining things lucidly. The CDC provided multiple updates throughout the day. All global brands, to begin with, and then our own Indian companies got into the act and solved the issues brilliantly. They provided us with the latest global technology and trained us quickly. Application specialists worked along with us. Indian companies were competing to provide global quality. There has been a large array of tests introduced, and we also have the technologies to do some of them. But RT-PCR has remained the gold standard for this test. We have also launched antibody tests for COVID-19. We are in the process of a tie-up with the IIT KGP (Indian Institute of Technology, Kharagpur), who have come up with a new methodology of testing COVID. And then we had the exposure to best practices from the leading academic institutes. In this ICMR played a grand role by continually publishing relevant data and answering queries. We ourselves have internal group discussions and have already hosted a couple of webinars on the same.

5. AH: Some tests could be expensive for the patients. How do you balance your responsibility as a medical professional, an owner of a lab facility, and as a civil society member in the middle of a pandemic of epic proportions?

SC: Yes, very much so. It takes expensive equipment, reagents, and highly qualified manpower to do the tests. But the industry rose to the occasion and very quickly rates were brought down, that actually enabled us to do this test at Rs 500 (about US$7) in one state.

We have been very clear about this and were the first to reduce prices. As a lab, we have tried the very best to provide quality. Besides, we've seriously invested in building QC within the lab.

Well, I think you need support from every corner to fight this pandemic. Very important at this stage is vaccination. There must be an elaborate plan to vaccinate 40–60 crore (400–600 million) people. That would need 1.2 billion doses of vaccine. The rich should try to help the poor.

6. AH: How did you balance the COVID-related tests and the non-COVID tests to maintain financial viability?

SC: The routine lab lost almost 60% of its regular mark. And that was that. No way were we going to see more number of patients. The COVID-19 business covered almost 50% of our losses at some stage. So, end-of-year books did not look that bad.

7. AH: Can the lab business make profits at times even in the midst of this pandemic? How do you balance profitability with corporate social responsibility in such troubled times?

SC: That is so true. But then whether you do it or not it is an ethical call that every organization has to take. We did PCR tests at the lowest possible rate. We will do vaccinations also at the lowest possible rate. We consider this to be the time when we have to contribute from the front. We are doing it.

PART III

HUMANITY IN PANDEMIC

Human Elements in a Crisis

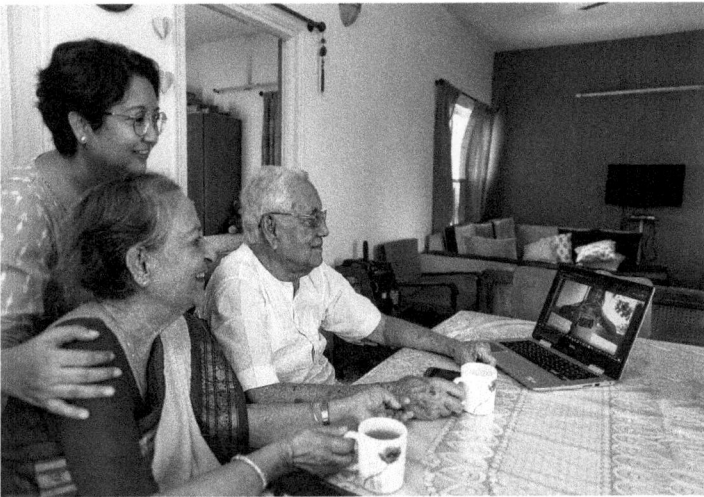

12

A FAMILY LAWYER'S OBSERVATIONS ON LIFE IN THE TIMES OF CORONAVIRUS

Kalyan Bhaumik

It is a melancholic aspect of my occupation that divorce cases comprise a significant part of my legal practice. As I am not qualified to be a therapist, my services to clients entail legal, not psychological, counselling, though many clients in adversarial family law cases are clearly suffering. Yet, as a social observer of many marriages in strife, I have noticed that certain patterns of attitudes and interactions of couples often determine troubled marriages are ultimately saved or doomed. Here though, I would like to make a couple of preliminary remarks on the short-term impact of the COVID crisis on the conjugal life of pre-separation stage couples in my city. My anecdotal evidence is derived from confidential telephone conversations with my clients who have seriously considered a mutual consent divorce but are still sharing the same roof with their spouses and who have kept me sporadically informed of the evolving interpersonal dynamics of their rarely placid home life. Naturally, I cannot disclose any facts that might reveal the specific circumstances of my clients. Nor is it possible to predict the effects of shared quarantine on failing marriages. But I will point out the signs of positive change in relationships that make me hopeful of the prospects of at least a few such marriages.

The most consequential effects of coronavirus are the lives lost to the contagion and the economy dislocated by the lockdown, but its most manifest effect is arguably the mildly adverse psychological

DOI: 10.4324/9781003218807-16

reaction of most people to enforced social isolation within the confines of their homes. Many millions are compelled to embrace temporarily an existence of uncertainty and immobility, and thus one of anxiety and boredom. Against this background of a worldwide public health crisis, countless individual households afflicted with marital discord are undergoing their own unique personal crises. Few would disagree with the second part of the famous opening sentence in Tolstoy's *Anna Karenina*: "All happy families are alike; each unhappy family is unhappy in its own way." Each breakdown of marriage has its own tragic narrative, yet sociologists, marriage counsellors, and divorce lawyers do recognize a few common themes in distressed marriages. One may assume that the various concurrent, novel stressors of life during this pandemic have combined to exacerbate marital tensions and dysfunction, especially during home confinement in the lockdown. But I have found that in more cases than not, the opposite is true in that the quality of marriage has actually improved a little since episodes of spousal conflict have become both less frequent and less intense, though the underlying issues of conflict may have been unresolved. In a minority of cases, however, I have found fragile marriages crumbling sooner than expected as some couples are coping poorly with the hardships of social isolation. Far from, a few of my clients cannot wait long enough for the lockdown to end to physically separate from their spouses.

What differentiates housebound couples who are moving closer towards divorce from those who are managing to coexist better? I have two small observations to make here. First, whether the quarantine is making bad marriages worse largely depends often on whether at least one of the two spouses has certain specific personality traits. Borrowing the parameters from the widely accepted Big Five Personality Traits model (McRae and Costa, 1987; Fetzer, 2021), I have observed in my rather small sample size of clients that almost invariably where at least one spouse has a high degree of neuroticism, even when the other spouse is of the "agreeable" type or is otherwise positive-thinking and not much antagonistic, the marriage has deteriorated precipitously during the COVID crisis. Psychologists variously describe a neurotic individual as worrying, nervous, high-strung, insecure, self-conscious, self-pitying, vulnerable, temperamental, impatient, jealous, and so forth. Such a subject is usually tense, moody, and irritable, often at once angry and depressed, and derives a low satisfaction from marriage. Being emotionally unstable and highly reactive to routine stressors, neurotic persons are often ill-equipped to handle the frustrations of enhanced stress during the quarantine that would demand greater resilience and adjustment. Irrespective of whether the neurotic person is my own client or my client's spouse (or rarely, both), with all other factors remaining the same, the discontent and volatility generated by the neurotic during the social isolation are destroying already strained marriages.

Second, whether spouses have been able to make life in their difficult marriages easier or at least more tolerable during the quarantine depends significantly on whether both spouses have proactively taken at least one of two measures to reduce or contain the damage. Empirically, such improvement has not resulted from any resolution of core differences, clearance of misunderstandings, better communications, family mediation, reciprocal compromises, unilateral appeasement, or emotional reengagement. For my clients, the two most effective moves to avert an imminent separation have been to reduce the mutual exchange of blame, and much more essentially, to mostly eliminate sarcasm in any form. This outcome confirms the findings of one of the foremost American researchers on the psychology of marriage, Dr John Gottman, who has identified criticism and contempt among the "Four Horsemen of the Apocalypse", his metaphor for the top four predictors of divorce (Lisitsa, 2021a,b). Criticism, when personal and not constructive, is not merely a complaint against someone's acts, but reflects one's disapproval of the other's character. Instead of inducing the other to change behaviour, disparagement serves only to widen any existing rift. But far more embittering is contempt, which is an assertion of one's moral superiority over the other conveyed through disrespect and callousness. It is the insult, subtle or otherwise, more than heated arguments, that devalues and scars the other permanently and is fatal to any relationship. The quarantine has afforded many people the opportunity to become a bit more self-aware of their own biases and triggers, preferences, and habits. Those few among my clients who have some common sense, good will, or whatever other motivation or impulse, largely refrained from showing contempt and moderated their criticism, are reporting greater satisfaction and lesser turbulence in their marriages. None can tell now in how many cases these very necessary changes would alone prove sufficient to preserve the marriage.

But some clients are already somewhat optimistic of their marriages despite challenges still to overcome. A few have told me that, while they appreciate my services, they feel encouraged to give their marriages another chance or two or three, so they will not proceed towards separation and divorce forthwith. On my part, I would happily lose them as satisfied clients and gain them as contented acquaintances instead.

NOTE

This contributed chapter was accepted for publication in this refereed edited volume on June 28, 2021.

REFERENCES

Fetzer, (2021), https://fetzer.org/sites/default/files/images/stories/pdf/self-measures/Personality-BigFiveInventory.pdf.

Lisitsa, E., (2021a), The Four Horsemen: The Antidotes, *The Gottman Institute*, 23 April 2021 https://www.gottman.com/blog/the-four-horsemen-recognizing-criticism-contempt-defensiveness-and-stonewalling/.

Lisitsa, E., (2021b), The Four Horsemen: Criticism, Contempt, Defensiveness, & Stonewalling, *The Gottman Institute*, 26 April 2021, https://www.gottman.com/blog/the-four-horsemen-recognizing-criticism-contempt-defensiveness-and-stonewalling/.

McCrae, R. and P. Costa, 1987, Validation of the Five-Factor Model of Personality across Instruments and Observers, *Journal of Personality and Social Psychology*, 52(1), pp. 81–90.

13

NO ONE CAN BE SAFE UNTIL EVERYONE IS SAFE

Sunanda K. Datta-Ray

The world is on the move. Death walks alongside as in Ingmar Bergman's film, *The Seventh Seal*. Sometimes Death masquerades as a monk, sometimes he cheats at chess to winkle out the winning move from Antonius Block, the knight whose search for a meaning to the riddle of life prompts an endless flow of questions. "Don't you ever stop asking?" Death demands as the spectral procession traipses through a plague-ravaged landscape. "No. I never stop" Block retorts. "But you're not getting an answer!" is Death's implacable reply.

Nevertheless, a glimpse of the answer to the larger and more vital question beyond the plague does emerge from the nature of the sickness. It is that man does not walk alone. Whether or not the pandemic has "changed forever the way we live our lives"—as an overwhelming 82 per cent of Britons polled by the national morning newspaper *I* agreed—the spectre of annihilation that is implicit in the pandemic is a stern reminder that despite raucous frictions, the world is one. Mankind's destiny is to stand or fall together.

The latest danger for COVID-19 patients—the agony of mucormycosis or the aggressive "black fungus"—is a reminder that the "All for One and One for All" motto of Alexandre Dumas's *The Three Musketeers* is the only recipe for survival today.

The World Health Organization (WHO) proclaimed a pandemic on 11 March 2020. The United States blamed the Chinese. China

DOI: 10.4324/9781003218807-17

denounced American participants in the Military World Games in the Wuhan province where it all began. Bats, chimpanzees, and pangolins, "the most illegally traded mammal in the world" according to the International Union for Conservation of Nature, were blamed. A tiger in a New York zoo was reportedly infected. No one knows for certain where the virus originated although the 120-page report by a WHO team that visited Wuhan suggests that it probably leapt from animals to humans through an emissary animal.

An early intimation of the fearsome news was the complaint in January 2020 of a 23-year-old Chinese national studying at Britain's York University who was suffering from fever, dry cough, and muscle pain. His 50-year-old mother, who had flown to Britain from Wuhan a week earlier, also had a fever, cough, and a sore throat. Coronavirus had spread by then to Thailand and the United States, with some 500 confirmed cases and 17 dead. That was the beginning. No one can be sure when—if ever—it will end. Or predict the devastation it might leave behind.

The threat is transboundary, as a minister in the Singapore government, Mohamad Maliki bin Osman, pointed out when the "Little Red Dot" made history by sending four cryogenic oxygen containers from Changi Airport to an airbase in West Bengal. More than 40 countries have since then poured lavish help into a stricken India whose pictures of the dead and dying, of coronavirus patients gasping for breath outside hospitals that were too packed to admit them, of cremation fires smouldering night and day, and the Ganges heavy with bloated corpses have gone viral on global television screens.

Things seemed so bad with government after government snapping travel links with India that friends thought my wife and me mad for returning after six months in London. We were moving from a cooling frying pan to a ferocious fire, they warned, quoting Delhi High Court's description of India's second wave as a tsunami. Wave or tsunami, it has been fanned by a number of factors. Official complacency, jubilantly rampaging cricket crowds, the Kumbh Mela festival when Hindus hope to wash away their sins in the holy Ganges (the *Hindustan Times* cited official sources to claim that 9.1 million pilgrims took the dip between 14 January and 27 April), Indian workers returning from abroad, Prime Minister Narendra Modi's *Tika Utsav* (Vaccination Festival) to cash in on the political legacy of anti-caste reformers, and the frenzy of fiercely fought elections in five states are blamed.

Infections reportedly increased tenfold in West Bengal where Modi's determination (unsuccessful as it happened) to capture the state for his Hindu majoritarian Bharatiya Janata Party made for an exceptionally bitter battle, especially when the Election Commission (EC, which organizes polls) overrode the state government's protests and insisted on protracted voting in eight phases. Inevitably, massive public rallies with Modi himself and his home minister, Amit Shah, putting in stellar appearances, ignored all pandemic protocols. Down South, the Madras High Court also blamed the EC, observing orally that it was "singularly responsible for the second wave of COVID" and that its officers "should probably be booked for murder".

Of course, the pandemic's trail of havoc is not confined to India. With its pockets of poverty and ethnic backwardness, the United States has fared worst. On his first day in office, President Joe Biden authorized action to halt construction of Donald Trump's controversial border wall, but could not wish away the crisis building up along the frontier with Mexico. The camps for hundreds of thousands of migrants seeking entry into the United States could be a breeding ground for COVID-19.

There were early signs of the staggering 4.3 per cent contraction of the global economy that economists predict. A devastating recession left 33 million Americans unemployed. At one point, every tenth person in London was jobless. The Pew Research Centre found that India's middle class shrunk by 32 million in 2020 while the daily earnings of 75 million Indians dwindled to $2 or less. While 10 million Chinese dropped out of the middle-income group, another 30 million fell into the low-income bracket of daily incomes ranging between $2.01 and $10. Since the two Asian giants account for more than a third of the world's population, these shifts are bound to affect global savings and spending.

Simultaneously, scarcities that lockdowns and closures compounded helped to line the pockets of resourceful operators, as in Britain during and after World War II when "spivs"—a new coinage then—made fortunes while law-abiding folk endured shortages and rationing. We cannot ignore the heroism of India's private volunteers or the dedicated service of underpaid and overworked doctors, nurses, and para-medical workers who are somehow coping with tremendous odds. Simultaneously, however, there are reports of oxygen cylinders stolen from legitimate users being sold on the black market. Of repainted fire extinguishers palmed off on the gullible as oxygen cylinders, and of funeral shrouds ripped from dead bodies peddled as new.

All prices are soaring—from country chicken to flights to New York, to say nothing of auto rickshaw fares to take COVID-19 victims to hospital. The New York Times News Service reports that ambulance drivers demand $70 (Rs 5,113) for the three-mile ride from hospital to cremation ground. Once there, firewood costs $70 instead of the normal $7 (Rs 513).

"Prosperity rules at the very top" *Forbes* proclaimed, noting "The three richest Indians alone have added just over $100 billion between them". *Forbes* also noted Mukesh Ambani "added nearly $48 billion to his fortune since last year, and reclaimed the title of Asia's richest person". India's then second richest—now the richest—billionaire, also with Gujarati roots like Ambani, infrastructure tycoon Gautam Adani, added $42 billion to his wealth.

Ironically, four of the wealthiest Indians are in healthcare. Cyrus Poonawalla whose Serum Institute of India, the world's largest vaccine manufacturer, makes Covishield, the Indian version of Oxford AstraZeneca, heads the pack. According to the Indian financial daily, *Mint*, he rents a mansion in London's Mayfair for a weekly $69,000.

Such linkages encourage rumours whose equivalent in Britain acquired something of the menace of Bergman's imagery. An ethnic Sylheti banker born and brought up in London's Brick Lane ghetto (immortalized in Monica Ali's eponymous novel) whispered that there was no pandemic, it was all a trick to deceive innocents. Hospital wards reserved for coronavirus patients lay empty, he said, while doctors were pressured to certify COVID-19 as the cause of death when people succumbed to other diseases. He hinted darkly that the British government collected a subsidy from some mysterious global entity for the number of coronavirus deaths it could show.

It was the opposite of India where the combination of suspected suppression, inadequate assessment, and ignorance is blamed for gross understatement of casualties. Few Indians are disposed to accept the official statistics of 26 million infections and just over 291,000 deaths—behind only the United States—by the third week of May. It is argued that even without deliberate fudging, there are few means of accurate assessment in remote villages where all illness is dubbed "bemaari", fever.

The American *QAnon* mystery is far more macabre with its symbol of a coiled serpent viciously poised to strike above the caption "Where we go one we go all". The British Broadcasting Corporation says, "At its heart, QAnon is a wide-ranging, completely unfounded theory that says that President Trump is waging a secret war against elite Satan-worshipping paedophiles in government, business and the media".

All crises generate such tittle-tattle. As the *Straits Times* recalled on 19 April 2020, "rumours that the [Spanish] flu [epidemic] could be prevented by eating boiled pumpkins, potatoes and coriander caused the prices of these items to skyrocket". The same paper disclosed that during the "Singapore Flu Scare" of 1957, "gossip spread across Chinatown and Queenstown that the pandemic had been caused by 'radioactive fallout from Russian hydrogen bomb tests', which the university authorities pooh-poohed as 'utter nonsense'".

Other COVID-19 rumours of military takeovers, tanks in the streets, corpses piling up in "every ice-skating rink", and helicopters secretly spraying disinfectant took me back to 1970 when I returned to a doleful Calcutta after three years abroad. Every street corner bustled with makeshift altars, coins were scattered on trays draped in red cloth, and few householders dared turn away persistent mendicants. A radical friend (Bengal bristled then with "champagne communists") who dismissed the paraphernalia as superstitious nonsense to placate the malefic Shani, Saturn, overlooked the sense of fear that underlies all propitiatory ritual.

A video titled *Plandemic: The Hidden Agenda Behind Covid-19* dangerously argues that vaccines are "a money-making enterprise that causes medical harm". Tapping into "people's uncertainty, anxiety and need for answers", its sequel, *Plandemic: Indoctrination* ("doctor" being highlighted in the logo to suggest indoctrination) echoed the nightmare vision of H.G. Wells's *The War of the Worlds* which was inspired by the brutal colonial subjugation of indigenous Tasmanians.

There are closer parallels. Shades of 1975 when Indira Gandhi's birth control campaign aroused the animosity of India's Gangetic peasantry, British canvassers plead that vaccination does not reduce fertility. Shades of the 1857 Indian Mutiny when fears of cow and pig lard being used to grease rifle cartridges alienated both Hindus and Muslims, the same canvassers insist that vaccines do not contain animal products. The emphasis during Ramadan was on denying there is any nutrient in vaccines. None of this fully allays the "vaccine hesitancy/resistance" of 31 per cent of Britain's population and 35 per cent of Ireland's which was especially regrettable in light of competing nationalisms and the European Union boycott of Astra-Zeneca despite the European Medicines Agency's categorical assertion that the vaccine's successes in preventing COVID-19 "outweigh the risks of side effects".

The economic rationale for hesitancy applies even more to India's cruel contrast of grinding poverty and ostentatious opulence with Mukesh Ambani paying £57 million during the pandemic for an estate in England, according to the *Times of India*. Britain's Bame (Black and Minority Ethnic) communities are sceptical about vaccination because being victims of "structural racism", they cannot benefit fully from social institutions and facilities. Statistics show that a black Briton is 70 per cent more likely than a white to live in a deprived area that suffers from pollution, congestion, and poor housing with limited access to education and employment. Most of these handicaps are aggravated in rural India where 70 per cent of Indians live. They are worst for the 364 million people (28 per cent of the population) languishing below the poverty level, according to the United Nations. They are at the mercy of a callously fragile health infrastructure.

Everything, not just oxygen, is in desperately short supply. India needs medicines, equipment, and hospital beds. Indian billionaires can hop into their private jets and whizz off to Geneva for a dentist's appointment, but the poor are stranded between the devil of ill-equipped, badly staffed, and negligent public hospitals and the deep of private institutions run by extortionate businessmen. India's 1.7 nurses per thousand people is well short of the WHO-recommended three-per-thousand. Although Indian doctors sustain Britain's National Health Service and many emigrate to the United States, the country's doctor-population ratio of 0.77:1,000 lags behind even China's 1.49 per thousand.

Yet, despite drawbacks, India, too, lived up to its moniker of pharmacy of the world by supplying close to 60 million doses to nearly 70 countries by the end of March 2021. Bharat Biotech co-developed Covaxin with the Indian Council of Medical Research, in addition to Poonawalla's Covishield. Modi obliged Trump by easing export restrictions on hydroxychloroquine, 70 per cent of global stocks being manufactured in India.

In contrast, some messages exchanged between Britain and her former EU partners recalled Carl von Clausewitz's definition of "war … by other means". Belgian officials raided AstraZeneca's production site near Brussels, the Dutch authorities seized ham sandwiches (unauthorized meat exports!) from British truck drivers, and British Foreign Secretary Dominic Raab accused the European Commission president, Ursula von der Leyen, of "brinkmanship".

Pestilences are a recurring phenomenon. Europe's 17th century plague, when Samuel Pepys noted the doleful call of "Bring out your dead!" and a red cross was chalked on infected houses with the legend, "Lord have mercy upon us", killed 25 million people. The Spanish Flu caused more than 50 million deaths. France's 19th-century cholera pandemic wiped out nearly 3 per cent of Parisians in a month.

Such terrors seldom start with a bang. Visiting Shanghai and Beijing in 2002, we were inclined to dismiss locals sporting face masks as faddists. A few months later, SARS (severe acute respiratory syndrome) was identified as a viral disease that had spread across the Pacific to Canada, the first severe and readily transmissible new disease to emerge in the 21st century. But the "race against death" that Britain's Iraq-born vaccine minister, Nadhim Zahawi, spoke of did not begin until the far more deadly strain of the virus was identified as severe acute respiratory syndrome coronavirus 2 (Sars-CoV-2).

This can be termed the bleak offside of the $2.9 trillion that travel and tourism earned in 2019. Not surprisingly, the United States accounted for the lion's share, an impressive $580.7 billion. But before the pandemic reduced the tiny former Portuguese enclave of Macau to a ghost town, it boasted the world's highest travel and tourism revenue as a share of gross domestic product.

Travel also includes foreign remittances. India led the list in 2019 when 17.5 million workers abroad repatriated $83.1 billion. China followed with $68.4 billion. With so much coming and going, it isn't surprising that India's second wave was most pronounced on the west coast which sends large contingents of workers abroad. Whether victims of war, political persecution, sectarian repression,

or racist pogroms like Myanmar's Rohingyas, the 79.5 million forc-
ibly displaced persons worldwide by the end of 2019 (8.7 million
more than the previous year) also demonstrated through their priva-
tions and hardships that the world is one. Each statistic set a dismal
record as countries struggled against a virus for which there was no
known cure until 19 March 2020 when the global pharmaceutical
industry announced a major commitment to address the challenge.

Several vaccines have been developed and marketed since then.
Several countries have shut down more than once. Britain declared
a lockdown on 23 March 2020. India followed two days later.
Although some restrictions have been eased since then, concerns
over slow vaccination, doubts about their efficacy, the emergence of
new and highly transmissible variants of the virus, political and
administrative disputes, and distractions like Modi's $2.8 billion
extravaganza to redesign New Delhi impede the smooth and stream-
lined campaign that India desperately needs.

While vaccination must be universal until herd immunity has
been attained, and there is no question of dispensing with sophisti-
cated medical treatment, prevention is said to be the most effective
response. Physical distancing and the basic rules of hygiene like not
spreading germs through spitting or sneezing, maintaining a safe distance between individuals, and regularly washing one's hands are
essential. India's vast numbers and the only lifestyle the multitude
can afford present the authorities with a daunting challenge. As
Nepal's plight tragically highlights, it's the same in all low-income,
semi-literate societies.

While they are not more likely to get coronavirus, they are more
likely to die if they do get it because the undernourished already
often suffer from chronic ailments.

The poor need more, not less, help. Incongruously, India spends
only 1.28 per cent of its gross domestic product on health against 2.4
per cent on defence. Rishi Sunak, Britain's ethnic Indian Chancellor
of the Exchequer, whose wife is the daughter of Indian IT tycoon
N.R. Narayana Murthy and is reputedly richer than Queen
Elizabeth, has cut overseas aid, compounding suffering in war-torn
South Sudan and Yemen.

The threat is not confined to any single group. It goes far beyond
John Donne's metaphysical vision of inter-dependence in the great
cycle of life and death. One coronavirus death does not only

diminish mankind; it threatens the entire human race with extinction. As Partha P. Majumder, president of the Indian Academy of Sciences and the West Bengal Academy of Science and Technology, wrote in *The Telegraph* newspaper of Calcutta, the only safety lies in a future "when no infected individual can find another individual to infect". That will not be possible until all individuals, especially in the world's most populous countries, are whole and healthy. Only then might the dirge of *The Seventh Seal* be defeated. We must live until then with the possibility that India's today could be the world's tomorrow.

NOTE

This contributed chapter was accepted for publication in this refereed edited volume on June 28, 2021.

JUDICIARY AND THE PANDEMIC

Debangsu Basak

Being largely ensconced in the legal fraternity for a major part of my life, my idea of the word "pandemic" was limited to the world of science fiction novels and movies.

The first coronavirus case in India was confirmed in Thrissur, Kerala, on 30 January 2020. The World Health Organization declared the coronavirus pandemic on 31 January 2020, as a global emergency of international concern. Slowly, but surely, the ramifications of the word "pandemic" began to sink in. The press and the social media brought the grim reality of the pandemic home.

In order to tackle the menace of the pandemic, most countries worldwide deployed lockdowns as a tactic. India, too, declared lockdowns. Initially, the lockdown was strict in the sense that movement of persons as well as vehicular traffic were restricted. The strict lockdown regime and its implementation resulted in a paradigm shift of the functioning of the courts in India.

Access to justice is one of the basic features of the Indian Constitution. The pandemic was affecting the fundamental right of the citizens of India to have access to justice. Like all other fields in the society, the pandemic caught the Indian judiciary not to be optimally prepared to tackle the menace. The Indian judiciary had to evolve measures and methods to overcome the unprecedented situation emanating out of the declaration of lockdown and the constitutional requirement to facilitate access to justice for the citizens.

DOI: 10.4324/9781003218807-18

During the initial period of the lockdown, with resources being scarce and unavailable, keeping the courts functioning was a Herculean task. The judiciary was required to strike a balance between safety of the personnel manning the judicial process and providing as unimpeded access to justice as possible in the prevailing lockdown norms.

Technology came to the rescue in dealing with the emergent situation emanating out of the declaration of a lockdown and the requirement to have access to justice. The courts migrated from physical hearing to virtual mode. This migration, however, was with its attendant share of challenges. Requisite infrastructure to hold courts virtually was not available at the optimum level and at the desired locations. The lack of infrastructure was both on account of unavailability of software and hardware. Internet facilities were not available with the requisite bandwidth to accommodate the quantum of traffic which a virtual court would require. The court administration grappled with the problem of having a software which was safe, secure, and easily accessible to all stakeholders; it would be compatible with available hardware and would be easy to navigate.

In order to overcome restrictions on movement, and to ensure minimal footfall in the court buildings, judges commenced holding courts from their residence. Stakeholders participating in the judicial process were allowed to participate in the court proceedings from the respective places where they were comfortable. They were not required to travel the distance to the court rooms to have access to justice. The number of courts in the virtual platform was reduced so as to strike a balance between the strict lockdown norms and the constitutional mandate of facilitating access to justice, under all circumstances. Again, with such an objective in view, the number and nature of court proceedings to be dealt with by the courts was also regulated.

The Supreme Court of India exercised powers under Articles 141 and 142 of the Constitution of India in a writ petition instituted by the Supreme Court Suo Moto being Suo Moto Writ Petition (Civil) No. 3 of 2020 where the Supreme Court extended the period of limitation for filing proceedings in a court of law in India.

The Supreme Court by its order dated 23 March 2020 passed in Suo Moto Writ Petition (C) No. 1/2020 In Re: Contagion of COVID 19 Virus in Prison constituted a High-Powered Committee comprising the Chairman of the State Legal Services Authority, the Principal Secretary (Home/Prison) and the Director-General of Prison to determine which class of detainees can be released on parole or on interim bail, for such periods as may be thought appropriate. This measure was put in place to decongest the correctional homes to some extent, without compromising the security of the society.

The Calcutta High Court passed an order on 24 March 2020, exercising powers under Articles 226 and 227 of the Constitution of India, extending the time period for all matters in which interim orders were subsisting as on 16 March 2020, and which may have expired, or which were due to expire on or before 19 April 2020. This extension was continued over a period of time. These orders of the Supreme Court and of the Calcutta High Court lengthened the time period for a litigant to approach the court. This extended time period released the pressure on a large section of the litigants to approach the court. It resulted in the salutary effect of lessening the footfalls at the court premises, protected the litigants, and at the same time gave relief with regard to the laws of limitation.

The Calcutta High Court also from time to time regulated the working of the court, both for the High Court and for the district judiciary, so as to prevent the spread of the virus and consequent loss of life. With the objective of minimizing the footfall at the court premises, the High Court as well as the district courts migrated from holding physical courts to holding courts on a virtual platform. This migration came with its attendant challenges. All stakeholders were not adequately trained for a seamless migration. Petitions were allowed to be filed online. The advocates were heard by the judges on the virtual platform. The courts were linked with the correctional homes, therefore negating the requirement of producing the accused physically before the court.

The Indian judicial system, howsoever stressed it may have become under the onset of the pandemic, has nonetheless stood up to the challenges and through an ongoing process of modulating its affairs to meet the emerging situations, is continuing to dispense justice.

The pandemic may have highlighted the inequality in the society on the socio-economic fronts. However, so far as access to justice and justice dispensation are concerned, the pandemic has permitted a much more widespread use of technology for the justice delivery ecosystem to penetrate to the lowest strata in the society. e-Sewa Kendras have been set up at district and High Court premises so that any person can approach the court on the virtual platform. The courts have mobilized requisite manpower to assist all stakeholders including the judges to conduct courts on the virtual platform.

The dissemination of information on social media and the bane of misinformation existed prior to the onset of the pandemic was further accentuated. The misuse and abuse of information on social media have to be dealt with through the existing laws and, if necessary, by a review of the existing system as well as the laws.

With the pandemic easing, the lockdown norms began to be relaxed gradually. The relaxation in the lockdown norms was availed of so as to broaden the reach of the judiciary in the justice dispensation ecosystem. More courts became functional. The courts strived to return to full-fledged functioning. The new normal, however, was required to be factored in with regard to the functioning of the courts. With such relaxations in place, the courts commenced with both physical as well as virtual hearings. The courts are presently continuing with the hybrid system of hearing.

Virtual courts are not without any drawbacks. Filings of voluminous documents are not unknown in court proceedings. The virtual platform is a quagmire for navigating documents without the requisite training. All stakeholders were not optimally trained to handle such situation with the onset of the pandemic. The economic condition of every litigant also could not be lost sight of. Every litigant may not be economically or otherwise empowered to avail of the virtual platform to have access to justice. There are, of course, issues in relation to the safety and security of the software used to facilitate the virtual court. Virtual courts will affect the existing system of a junior lawyer developing his skills through assisting a senior lawyer in court in the physical format. However, a junior lawyer with requisite drive will adapt to the present system and learn his skills on the new platform.

So far as litigations are concerned, an original proceeding requires evidence to be taken both in the criminal as well as in civil jurisdictions. A trial in a criminal case requires oral evidence to be taken, experts to be examined, and in certain cases materials to be exhibited. The virtual platform is not well suited for conduct of such type of cases. The Indian judiciary is evolving various norms and methods to overcome the challenges of dealing with original proceedings where evidence and particularly oral evidence is required to be adduced. Witness demeanour is one of the important facets in oral evidence. Ideally oral evidence should be taken in the presence of the judge deciding the *lis* (legal dispute) and in a court physically. The virtual platform does not highlight the witness demeanour which a court held physically would.

The challenges of having courts on the virtual platform are many but not insurmountable. With the passage of time and assistance of technology these challenges can be successfully overcome. Artificial Intelligence is one field which the judiciary can explore for a more robust delivery of justice in a time-bound manner and with desired exactitude. However, artificial intelligence has its own limitations.

However ghastly the pandemic panned itself out globally on the socio-economic front, it resulted in some positivity; these positives may be few and insignificant as compared to the negatives of the pandemic. The pandemic jolted the courts in India to migrate from physical hearing to the virtual platform. In utilizing the virtual platform, the courts were no longer limited within the geographical boundaries of the walls of the court rooms. It transcended such boundaries to travel right to the doorstep of the litigant seeking justice. In fact, it stepped into the arena of the litigant, at the choice of the litigant. The litigant was no longer required to travel the distance to the court so as to avail justice. Besides, the courts were able to meet the litigant at a place of the choice of the litigant so as to render justice. A court holding a physical hearing would be hard pressed to meet every litigant at a place of the choice of the litigant to deliver justice.

The pandemic has allowed the judiciary to innovate and experiment. It has allowed the judiciary to take assistance of available technology at a scale which was momentous. The pandemic has established the relevance of technology in the judicial field. It has gone a long way to promote a better integration of technology with the existing structure of justice dispensation. Aid and assistance of technology in the justice delivery system has been appreciated more than before. It has accelerated the integration of technology in the justice delivery ecosystem. The need to evolve and implement technological tools so as to make justice available to the person needing it, at a place where such person is comfortable to receive it, is being appreciated and worked upon. Over a period of time, surely, a more seamless integration of technology with the justice dispensation system will result in an improved quality of justice being delivered to the doorstep of the litigant seeking justice.

The pandemic has allowed the Indian judiciary to evolve in unprecedented ways. Many changes ushered in are likely to stay.

NOTE

This contributed chapter was accepted for publication in this refereed edited volume on June 26, 2021.

COVID-19 AND MICRO, SMALL, AND MEDIUM ENTERPRISES

Many Misses, Some Hits

Anurag Srivastava

In the first fortnight of January 2020, the World Health Organization (WHO) reported a new type of pneumonia that was spreading in China from the novel coronavirus. By 21 January 2020, when the WHO published its first situation report, there were 282 confirmed cases of this new illness named COVID-19, three of them outside China. After that the situation unfolded rapidly, and pictures of scores of patients on ventilator support and hundreds of daily deaths, emanating first from Italy and then from many other countries, shook the world. In the collective memory of mankind, what happened afterwards is etched clearly. There were lockdowns across countries with cities wearing deserted looks and everything came to a standstill. The exponential curves forecasting future case load/deaths predicted doom. Never before had the world faced a crisis of this magnitude, and each country was bracing itself for an impending avalanche of COVID-19. On 11 March 2020, the WHO declared it a pandemic, and by this time COVID-19 had entered 114 countries. As per the WHO dashboard on 6 September 2020, there were 26,763,217 confirmed cases of COVID-19 and 876,616 deaths due to it.

The idea of this chapter is not to discuss further what has been mentioned above, but to look at the impact of COVID-19 on Micro, Small and Medium enterprises (MSMEs). MSMEs consist of

DOI: 10.4324/9781003218807-19

micro units which may be single-person enterprises, small units which may be of reasonable size, and medium units having many employees. The experience presented in the chapter is from West Bengal, a state of India on the eastern side. West Bengal has almost 9 million MSMEs which employ more than 13 million people. Most of the MSMEs of West Bengal are small one-member units. The objective of this chapter is to look at the onset of COVID-19 and related actions due to it, particularly the effect of lockdown on MSMEs. This chapter will mostly try to look at the human aspect of the impact, and if things could have been done differently. We are still not in a position to assess the complete impact of COVID-19, but a lot has happened, from the beginning of strict lockdowns to unlocking the economy, and the story of MSMEs deserves to be told.

The first case of COVID-19 was detected in the state of West Bengal on 17 March 2020. Different restrictions were imposed during that period by the state governments, like closing of schools and restriction on gatherings. On 22 March 2021, the Prime Minister called for 'Janta Curfew' or 'voluntary lockdown' for 14 hours, and this became a precursor for a complete lockdown from 24 March 2020. This lockdown was announced by the Prime Minister Mr Narendra Modi on live TV at 8 PM on 23 March and was made effective from midnight. Not much time was given for preparation as it appeared that the idea was to have an element of surprise and ensure everyone stays where s/he is. Like most activities, a business enterprise does not have a button to turn it on and off. A business activity runs in a cycle, and there are consequences of stopping it in between. There were furnaces that needed time to be closed properly, there was raw material stocked, but most of all, there were workers at the sites, many of whom came from far off places. It may not be wrong to say that the situation was chaotic. The focus of the administration was to enforce complete lockdown, and everything was closed in panic. The strict lockdown that began for 21 days ultimately got stretched beyond 45.

It may be wrong to put the entire blame for the chaos that ensued on the government. The exponential rise in cases and mortality rate in the initial phase of COVID-19 and the factor of unknowns demanded urgent action. There was widespread panic, and many countries had started lockdowns. The health set-up was not yet prepared and needed time to gear up for this challenge. The lock-down order did allow exceptions like permitting enterprises associ-ated with essential items or production units that needed continuous process. Most of these exemptions, however, remained on paper as there was no clarity which essential items would be allowed to con-tinue. Adding to that there is a complete ecosystem and supply chain that works for any industry, and unless all of them are allowed, indi-vidual units cannot function. For example, food items were exempted, but not the packaging industry, and the former cannot run when the latter is closed. Even for units which opened, there was the issue of transportation of workers. There was no public transport, and even if units could arrange private transport, no one knew how passes and permissions were to be issued. There was lack of clarity, but the priority of the government was to tackle the emerging health situation, rather than assist the industry. Also, due to the general lockdown, government offices were closed. They were running with skeleton staff, and this impacted decisions and overall functioning. Thus, as the lockdown began from 25 March 2020, there was a total shutdown in the industry.

Soon it dawned that everything cannot remain closed. For some days before the actual lockdown, there was panic buying, and it appeared there may be shortages of essential items during the lock-down. There was also an emerging demand for personal protective equipment (PPE) for the health sector, and with the ban on free movement items were to be locally supplied. A group of senior officers of the government was designated to get industries started on a case-by-case basis and issue necessary clarifications. Mechanisms were devised to issue different permissions with the use of information technology (IT) to streamline the process. There were restrictions that were imposed on industries which were allowed to function. Most of them were asked to run with 50% or less workforce. Strict conditions were laid down like com-pulsory wearing of mask, mandatory provision of handwashing, and maintaining of social distancing. The timing of running these units was fixed, and such units were allowed only in regions with no active cases.

The industries which got permission to operate faced many diffi-culties. They faced resistance from the inhabitants of the neighbour-hood where they were located. Locals feared these industries could end up bringing COVID-19 to their localities. Workers who worked in these industries found it difficult to commute as there was no transport. Apart from the government-enforced lockdown, a concept of 'para lockdown' meaning 'community lockdown' was enforced which meant people belonging to a neighbourhood decided amongst themselves that no outsider would be allowed to enter, and anyone who goes outside would not be allowed to return. These local restrictions were so strong that even the disposal of the dead body of COVID-19 patients became a headache for the administration as people did not allow crematoriums located in their area to be used for cremating dead bodies of people who were not residents of that locality. These local restrictions meant anyone staying in such places could not go out to work even if exempted by the government.

A big impact of COVID-19 on the industry was the disruption in the supply of workers. As per some estimates, there are roughly 120 million migrant workers in India. These people leave their homes in search of better opportunities often leaving their families behind. In many industries, skilled labour comes from specific regions. Industries also prefer to employ workers from outside because they come cheap, do not cause local trouble, and are reliable in not claiming unexpected leave. Few of them enjoy job security, and their living conditions are far from satisfactory. These people were hit hardest due to COVID-19. When the lockdown started, many of them found themselves out of a job. Moreover, they could not move back to their homes due to the strict lockdown and restriction on transport. Although the government directed the industries to pay them wages, it was difficult to enforce such a directive. As days passed, hundreds of such workers started walking back towards their homes. They suffered innumerable hardships on the route, from being branded as carriers of COVID-19 to being prosecuted for not following government directives. Many of them walked for more than 1,000 kilometres and reached home walking 15–20 days. Different accidents claimed the life of more than 300 migrants. After the partition of India, this was the largest man-made exodus, and lockdown guidelines failed to address the plight of these migrants. When the process of unlocking the economy started, industries struggled to bring back these migrant workers. The psychological scars of this event will take a long time to heal.

An unintended consequence of COVID-19 was insulation of the economy. After World War II, it was the first time that the country's economy was cut off from outside. Not only was international trade hampered, even local movement of materials within the country became difficult. This resulted in demand exceeding supply, and local industries were expected to supply these items. It was also realized that the country depended on imports for many essential items, especially those needed by health fraternity for fighting COVID-19 like the PPE. This came as an opportunity for local MSMEs. A PPE suit creates a protective cover for the wearer preventing any transmission of virus from an infected person; it is impermeable to bodily fluids. Dungaree or the coverall, which is the most important part of the PPE suit, is a dress stitched from a specific material. The strength of an MSME is its ability to adapt, and MSMEs played this role well. With active support from the government, many units involved in the textile business started producing PPE coveralls. During the lockdown when their normal business was nil and there was no demand for their original product, they were more than eager to enter this business. The only assistance they needed from the government was technical know-how and quality parameters along with necessary permissions to operate during the lockdown. In the state of West Bengal, local MSMEs produced more than 2 million PPE suits in a span of four months along with more than 5 million masks. This business opportunity helped some MSMEs to do profitable business during this difficult time. Even in other items, MSMEs which got permission to operate did brisk business. Anecdotally, many industries shared that business was profitable during this period even though production was less because of increase in prices and transactions being done on upfront payment basis with no credit.

Despite these few areas where there was increased business opportunity, it was clear that the lockdown was having an adverse impact on the economy. The government did try to help. There were various interventions, and the government claimed these cumulatively amounted to roughly 10% of total GDP (rupees 20 trillion or $270 billion). Most of these were related to infusion of liquidity through measures like auto enhancement of existing credit limit or introducing schemes for infusion of credit through equity. Some long-term changes were also introduced by the government like changing the definition of MSMEs. There are many government schemes to promote MSMEs, and industries are classified as MSME based on their investment in plant and machinery and overall turnover. There had been a demand for revising the definition of MSMEs upwards, as earlier definition was more than a decade old. The definition of MSMEs was revised during this period, and applicable investment/turnover was increased by more than five times. Industries having an annual turnover up to rupees 250 crores ($35 million) were now eligible as an MSME. There was a specific thrust of the government to promote local industries. Besides, restriction was placed on inviting global tenders for contracts less than rupees 200 crores ($27 million). Prime Minister Mr Narendra Modi, during this period, had a slogan 'Vocal for Local,' i.e. active promotion of local industries.

After 75 days of strict lockdown, the Government of India started what was called 'Unlock 1' on 8 June 2020. The idea was to ease restrictions gradually and restart the economy. Till 30 September 2020, guidelines of 'Unlock 4' were applicable in India, and still there were various restrictions. While industries were being reopened in a gradual manner, there were reports of more than 30 serious industrial accidents that killed 75 people and injured 100 others. There were incidents of poisonous gas leaks, boiler explosions, and fire. It was apparent that these were the result of industries being halted without a proper shutdown process. Adding to that, inspection and maintenance of industrial units suffered during this period, resulting in accidents. This was a factor that was ignored while planning and implementing the lockdown.

When the lockdown began, there was a glimmer of hope that we could restrict the COVID-19 virus by remaining closed for some days. Soon it was clear that was not going to be the case, and the lockdown could never have been a permanent solution. Slowly countries have started to reopen, but there is a 'new normal' everywhere. The market today is different from the one that existed before, and demand of products has undergone change. While people are buying more items, many sectors are witnessing a decline. People are still hesitant to venture out, and spending is on necessary items. During this period, there was a boom in e-commerce as it avoided physical contact. Thus, many industries are switching towards a digital medium, and technology is bridging physical barriers. There has been a big thrust in digital payments. Any change is also an opportunity for innovation, and many new ways to conduct business have arrived. It appears that MSMEs with capability of being on the right side of the digital divide will have a better chance to survive. Skilled workers are still not back from their native places, and industries are trying to find measures to woo them back. There are new opportunities due to thrust on local industries by the government, but there are challenges due to implicit/explicit barriers in imports. Industries are not sure if fluctuations in demand is temporary, or capital investments are worth during this period. There is further uncertainty of local lockdowns. COVID-19 cases in an area can make it a containment zone, inviting restrictions of lockdown.

The industry paid a heavy price for COVID-19 and lockdown, and there was 23.9% contraction in the gross development product (GDP) in the April–June quarter of 2020–2021 as per official statistics released by the National Statistical Office (NSO). Amongst large economies, the Indian economy fared the worst during this period. On the COVID-19 front, cases in India are yet to peak, with daily cases setting new record every day. As of 7 September 2020, India had overtaken Brazil and was the second worst hit country in the world, after the United States. New daily cases are nearing six digits, and soon we may have more than 100,000 cases in a day. India still has fared better in fatality rate and cases per million population, and it may be due to the strict lockdown.

With the benefit of hindsight, we can say some things could have been done differently. There is a point of view that says the lockdown in India was imposed too fast. It was also one of the strictest when compared to other countries. We probably assumed that with the strict lockdown for some days, COVID-19 would vanish. It was already too late, and the government took a long time to understand the restrictions, and COVID-19 would coexist for years, if not decades. India is a large and diverse country, and a better strategy could have been to define broad parameters and empower state and local governments to choose amongst different lockdown strategies. Something that works in a dense urban neighbourhood is not useful in sparsely populated villages and vice versa. The spread of COVID-19 was also different in different areas. If there was better communication defining the objective of lockdown, a flexible strategy could have been adopted at local government level that would have yielded similar results.

The government also failed to understand that restricting any movement is not only difficult to implement but also counterproductive. People could have been told in advance the strategy of the government to take them back to their native place, if they wanted to go. With each passing day increasing their restlessness and no clear communication from the government, migrants started walking on the roads resulting in an unnecessary loss of almost 300 lives. By 30 June 2020, there was almost 20% of COVID-19 deaths India had witnessed. These migrants walked like criminals avoiding authorities, and this increased the loss of life. For example, 16 migrants were crushed by a goods train when they were sleeping on a railway track at night because they chose to avoid roads and walked on railway tracks to evade the police who would have stopped them from going back. When the government realized it needed to make arrangements to ease their movement, most of the migrants had lost faith in the government and started moving back in hordes, at the first available opportunity.

Welfare orientation during the lockdown was also a reactive not a proactive strategy. Many of the economic measures introduced by the government to give impetus to industries were not started simultaneously with the lockdown. MSMEs employ more than 110 million people in India and contribute roughly 30% to India's GDP. Any lockdown that basically shuts down this sector should have had special ameliorating strategy for this sector.

As previously mentioned, a positive aspect of this lockdown was a push towards digitization. Units today are more comfortable in conducting their business through online medium, holding meetings through video conference, and taking orders through social media platforms. This has in a way given them a larger platform to showcase their products, and with the right kind of support, many MSMEs can attract national and international buyers. This can also give impetus in increasing exports from these units.

A part of the misery of MSMEs was brought by COVID-19, and a part of it was brought by the lockdown. For any government, this was the first experience with COVID-19, and it may be unfair to blame them completely for fallout of lockdowns, but we can learn. On the positive side, we can hope that the worst is over, and things can only improve from now on. On the negative side, India may be quite far from its peak load of COVID-19. The story is still unfolding, and let us hope that when we reach denouement, the ending is positive for the industry and MSMEs. In some ways, the opening paragraph of Charles Dickens' novel, *A Tale of Two Cities* comes to mind.

> It was the best of times, it was the worst of times, it was the age of wisdom, it was the age of foolishness, it was the epoch of belief, it was the epoch of incredulity, it was the season of light, it was the season of darkness, it was the spring of hope, it was the winter of despair.

NOTE

This contributed chapter was accepted for publication in this refereed edited volume on May 5, 2021.

BRIDGE OVER TROUBLED WATER
A CEO's Perspective on Navigating the Pandemic

Ajay Bhattacharya

INTRODUCTION

There is and will continue to be numerous challenges in our lives. These challenges can be broadly categorized as personal, national (country specific) or international (worldwide).

From your perspective, personal challenges are normally easier to handle when the world around you is calm. As you move from the realm of "personal" to "international," the complexities of the challenges tend to increase.

Let us consider some "what if" scenarios.

Just imagine if in the middle of your own personal challenge, the country you are in is also in turmoil. In such a scenario, you might even contemplate leaving your country for the safety and security of a more stable country. But what if the issue is global? Where do you fly to for safety? Unfortunately, in 2020, the world did have such an issue, and there was no country that was spared by the COVID-19 virus. You just could not fly out of your own country to be somewhere else, somewhere safe. How are you going to tackle a worldwide issue, particularly when your tools to tackle these challenges are limited?

When you cannot use existing tools to tackle the existing challenges, it is time to **change**.

DOI: 10.4324/9781003218807-20

The change can be in the form of mindset, habits, and daily living. We have to come up with new norms for both work and home. On a more personal note, I took the "change" approach for one big reason.

CHANGE IS THE ONLY CONSTANT IN LIFE: HERACLITUS: 535 B.C.

From a young child to an adult, we have had to change all the time: from a student to becoming a working adult, getting married, having kids, retiring, and the list goes on. Most people change when faced with crisis or a threat. Not many people change when things are going on smoothly.

I have taken this COVID-19 journey as I would do for anything else. From my perspective, the pandemic brought about by COVID-19 is a very dangerous event, and we have to accept it as it poses an existential threat. As with any threat, we must be able to deal with it and not ignore it. If we deal with it with respect, we will thrive, but if we ignore the destructive impact, we will perish. As a CEO and as a member of the civil society, we have done many things in order to navigate the challenges of COVID-19, since February 2020.

In this chapter, we will show that if we are agile and accept change, we will be able to thrive under any circumstance and not just COVID-19. We will start with how we had to change our modus operandi, ensuring that the business and livelihood of the staff and their family remain intact. Once livelihood is taken care of, we will then see how we continue to remain healthy under the lockdown. Finally, once we have successfully looked after ourselves, we can then look after society and show gratitude for our survival.

THE BEST WAY TO GET STARTED IS TO QUIT TALKING AND BEGIN DOING—WALT DISNEY

On February 7, 2020, the Singapore Government declared Disease Outbreak Response System Condition (DORSCON) code Orange. Under the DORSCON framework, orange means the outbreak is deemed to have moderate to high public health impact. The DORSCON code was set up after the Singapore SARS outbreak in 2003. Prior to the COVID-19 outbreak, it was used only once during the 2009 Swine flu 9 H1NI situation.

Upon realizing that the next stage would be DORSCON Red, the planning team did scenario planning and simulated what would happen during DORSCON Red. What was very concerning is the need for schools and offices to be closed for a period of time to contain and mitigate the transmission and impact. This would also imply that office workers, including the management team, will not be able to rush back to pick up documents and files from their respective offices, if needed.

FEBRUARY 15, 2020

First step we took was to set up the Business Continuity Plan (BCP) team who had come up with the plans for moving the office in its entirety to work from home (WFH) mode. The BCP team broke up the migration to WFH into several phases, to make it more functional. For example, we adopted following a contingency plan to deal with the crisis.

The company was divided into two teams (Team A and Team B); all department members are represented in both teams. For example, each team had personnel from Management, Commercial, Operations, Hedging, and Middle Office. This would ensure that each team can function on its own. In the first two weeks Team A did odd days (Monday, Wednesday) while team B did the even days (Tuesday, Thursday). We decided to get the full office in on Fridays following all safety management protocols.

The first two weeks of Phase 1 was a process of self-discovery. At the end of this initial phase, we had to identify:

a   Issues with Working from Home
b   Issues with Digitization.

We knew that most of the employees did not have any experience working from home. We also knew that they might not be able to work at home. That is the reason, to begin with, we did alternate days and not alternate weeks. This gradual deployment of the split-team arrangement allowed them to understand the limitations of working from home. They observed what was lacking and identified the Information Technology (IT) support they needed. The IT personnel also found out what the systems could handle and what needed to be upgraded.

One major point that we realized was that many staff did not have laptops as they worked exclusively in the office and had their desktops. Some of them also did not have Wi-Fi connections at home as they used their mobile phones to check emails after work.

Phase 2 was implemented once we had tackled most of the infrastructure issues. The teams were then made to do alternate weeks (instead of alternate days). This was the first time most of us had to work from home for an extended period. For instance, in my case I had to work from home for 2 weeks as my daughter had arrived from the United Kingdom and had to serve a 14-day Stay-Home Notice (SHN).

APRIL 7, 2021

Ultimately, by the time a Circuit Breaker (90% of DORSCON Red) was announced on April 3 and implemented on April 7, we had 6 weeks of training/practise; the entire office did not face any issues in adjusting to the new regulations.

THE NEW NORMAL

MTM (Management Teams Meeting)

For the first time in the existence of our company, we had a distributed workforce. The standard operating procedures (SOPs) in the company was based on the understanding that we would always be able to meet and discuss as a group.

With a distributed workforce, we needed to ensure the following:

a   All teams integrate and communicate with one another, and not only in their own team.
b   The documentation and approvals should have a proper flow.
c   There must be tighter controls as it was a distributed workforce.

In order to achieve the first two objectives, we set up 15 teams and conducted 15 MTMs per week. Many of the staff were involved in numerous teams, and there was always an overlap. This overlap ensures that we had cross-breeding of ideas and prevented silos from setting in.

To ensure that there was no collusion or cutting of corners, we implemented tighter controls and approvals involving several departments.

Any decision that was unanimous did not need the approval of the Managing Director. However, if there were any objections, we would call for a team meeting to discuss the objections and make a collective decision. This would then become an SOP. All new decisions taken were then compiled into an Operating Handbook for a distributed workforce.

INCREASED HEDGING ACTIVITY

In the beginning of 2020, the world was slowly being engulfed by COVID-19. The pandemic was spreading fast and furious. Our highly integrated and globalized society enabled diseases to spread very fast across borders. As the world went into lockdown, the markets became very volatile. By March 2020, we witnessed the largest stock market crash in history due to the pandemic and fear of recession. We took the view that this was only the beginning and things could get worse. We had to do something.

Up to now the team was empowered to be reactive, i.e. only do physical hedges. However, we had to be ahead of the market in a limited way, and we changed our rules of hedging to allow this.

The main aim of the hedging team was to prevent losses. We are a physical player in the petroleum and petrochemical market. We have feedstocks and production facilities. Therefore, we are always "long" in products. Since we are long, we need to make sure that in a downward market, we need to be ahead of the game. In that way, we can prevent a huge loss to prices of the existing products that we have.

By protecting our costs, we were not looking to make a profit when the market collapsed. This simple narrative (to prevent loss) ensured that the hedging team did not speculate the bottoming-out of the market. They did not speculate and were not allowed to speculate. This turned out to be a saving grace. At the end of April 2020, the crude market became negative and that forced many companies into insolvency.

With the change in internal controls, board approvals, and beefing up of the hedging teams, we managed to manoeuvre the highly volatile period.

TO SEE WHAT IS RIGHT, AND NOT DO IT IS A LACK OF COURAGE—CONFUCIUS

Many companies went into insolvency, and one of the largest in Singapore was Hin Leong with a loss of $4 billion. This happened in April 2020, while on lockdown which hit the Singapore banks very badly.

Banking and trade finance is the lifeblood of our business. We need banks and trade finance lines to do business. Since most of the banks in Singapore were hit, there might be a knee-jerk reaction forcing banks to review all clients.

As a result of this our management went into scenario planning, "What if we do not have trade lines?" We need to plan what business we should continue doing and what we can avoid doing in case the worst happens, i.e. banks freezing our lines. Essentially the commercial team and our offices worldwide were asked to speak to their customers. They could then identify which businesses were suffering and would most likely consume less chemicals. By working with our customers, we were able to identify less profitable businesses and therefore, work towards mutually agreeing to cancel the contracts.

As a result of taking this step we were able to keep the profitable deals and reduce the least profitable deals. Ultimately in June 2020, due to the Hin Leong issue, the banks did come down hard with all customers and cancelled 50% of the trade finance lines. While this did affect us, we were able to allocate the lines to deal with our existing profitable customers.

THE PESSIMIST SEES DIFFICULTY IN EVERY OPPORTUNITY. THE OPTIMIST SEES OPPORTUNITY IN EVERY DIFFICULTY—WINSTON CHURCHILL

From January 2020, when COVID had hit China, it was getting very difficult to run our refinery in Korea due to the delays in shipping. As a result, we decided to reduce the run rate of the factory. We took a proactive approach, i.e. informing our customers that we will not be supplying the finished goods. Our customers were then free to source from elsewhere.

Since we had taken the first-mover advantage, most of our customers appreciated us for being open and direct. They also had ample time to find alternatives.

In March 2020, we decided to stop the refinery keeping a minimal staff and sending most of the workers home. We continued to pay them so that they would be on standby to restart the refinery when the impact of the pandemic was over. In hindsight, that was the best decision we made as the market went for a free fall from the end of March, and we would have lost millions had we continued our operations. During the shutdown, we did more housekeeping and improvements in the refinery.

HEALTH AND WELL-BEING

During the lockdown people spent more time in their homes. They had access to healthy food in their own refrigerators, as they were the ones buying the food.

As gyms were closed, there was explosion of exercise apps. These apps were for all sorts of activities from running, body weights, yoga, and so on. A virtual coach would instruct you on what exercises you had to do. You also had physical fitness challenges, and results were compared to others in the virtual world. There were also numerous virtual marathons that you ran individually and uploaded the results online.

Due to the lockdown, we also had less air pollution from cars, planes, and factories, just to name a few. Cleaner air, healthier food, and lots of exercise provided the opportunity for people to become healthy. Also, for the first time many families stopped travelling and stayed indoors at home. It forced families to stay together and spend time talking and enjoying each other's company.

We have discussed how we managed the complexities and challenges by changing the way we operate. However, surviving is a raison d'être. The question was how do we do more than survive—and thrive?

THE HUMAN CONNECTION: GRATITUDE

It Is under the Greatest Adversity That There Exists the Greatest Potential for Doing Good, Both for Oneself and Others: Dalai Lama

Singapore has a large population (approx. 300,000) of workers living in dormitories. The Singapore Ministry of Manpower and the

Ministry of Health commented, "47 per cent of migrant workers in S'pore dorms have had a Covid-19 infection" (The Straits Times, December 15, 2020).

The worst cluster in Singapore was the foreign workers, many of whom were from Bangladesh. When you are sick you tend to miss home-cooked meals. They were getting meals from various people; however, what they longed for was Bengali dishes like fish curry, mixed vegetables (Shukto) and rice, and lentils (Dal/Bhat).

On April 14, 2020, Singaporeans received a $600 grant from the government as part of the solidarity payment. My wife Paramita wanted to donate this to charity. However, upon seeing the dorm workers in trouble and as a great cook herself, she decided to cook Bengali food to feed the dorm workers to their delight on Sunday May 24, 2020, on the auspicious occasion of Eid.

COVID-19 was a great educator. We learnt the hard way that we will need to respect nature more and in essence go back in time, where we stop sometimes to smell the roses, travel less, and more importantly spend more time with your loved ones.

NOTE

This contributed chapter was accepted for publication in this refereed edited volume on April 8, 2021.

VIRTUAL FIRESIDE CONVERSATIONS WITH PROFESSIONALS AND BUSINESS LEADERS

Advocate Kalyan Bhaumik (KB)

Conversation with **Dr Suborno Bose (SB), DBA, FCA, D. Edu, DSc. (Hon. Causa), on Leisure and Hospitality Industry**

Being an entrepreneur is second nature to Dr Suborno Bose, a Chartered Accountant, an educator, a hotel owner, and a business leader. He is the founder of the multinational Indismart Group Worldwide and is Chairman of the Indian Institute of Hotel Management (IIHM), India's premier international hospitality management institution. Dr Bose being the CEO of the International Hospitality Council finds himself in one of the hardest times for the industry that he dedicated his life to promote through education and training.

1 KB: How has the global pandemic affected the hospitality industry in India and globally?

SB: One of the worst hit industries in the world during the pandemic has been the hospitality industry. The hospitality industry is largely based on business travels, and due to the lockdown, there has been little or no business travels globally. As a result, globally, the industry recorded mammoth losses, both in terms of rooms sales, and

DOI: 10.4324/9781003218807-21

food and beverages sales. In India the industry suffered a major set-back, and the leisure hotels did some business only for a few months. Overall, the industry has incurred a loss of over Rs 130,000 crores (USD 17.9 billion) in 2020/2021, a decline of 75% as compared to 2019/2020. There was a decline of 38.7% in revenue per available room (RevPAR) during the first quarter of 2021 year on year in India.

2 KB: How has the education and training including job prospects changed in the industry?

SB: While the education and learning continued online and through digital medium, the job market had been bleak, and no hotels or restaurants were eager to recruit new employees. However, other sectors have recruited from the hospitality sector, like healthcare and hospitals.

3 KB: What are the potential catalysts of growth that you see in hospitality and travel industry in a post-pandemic world?

SB: We are looking at good economic boom post October 2021, with the second wave subsiding, and it seems that both the business hotels and leisure hotels would do much better than in 2020. New concepts like staycation, work from hotel, and home delivery of food and beverages has opened new avenues of revenue and profit. Domestic tourism would see a big boom as Indians will avoid travelling abroad till 2023 and will travel within the country.

4 KB: There are different innovations that came about due to the pandemic. Many hotels have collaborated with hospitals providing accommodation as quarantine facilities as well as for isolation or stay-at-home notices. Singapore airlines opened up their catering service to be available for dine-ins in their A380 planes on the tarmac. AirAsia started a food and other product delivery business to diversify their offerings. Do you foresee such bundling of products in future to preserve brand value or is it just a one-off due to the pandemic?

SB: The pandemic has opened many innovative strategies, and hotels as semi-hospitals and safe homes plus quarantine centres have become extremely popular. Such brand bundling would be an interesting thing to see in the near future.

5 KB: There has been discussion on centralized kitchens and just-in-time delivery options among different quarters. What do you foresee as innovation and digitalization for the industry?

SB: I think the industry has to depend on embracing technology to survive. Whether it's mobile phone–enabled room keys or cloud kitchen or deliver food in time with tech support, the technology is going to drive the future of hospitality.

6 KB: As an impact of the global pandemic, what changes do you see are permanent and what do you think are temporary in the hospitality industry in India and globally? What should hotel owners do to take on these new challenges?

SB: I think a lot will change in future permanently and with tech-heavy means. In the short run, the hotel owners have to make money through the pandemic-created opportunities. But overall, I think the hospitality industry will bounce back quite strongly at the end of 2021, and by 2022 it will come back to normalcy.

NOTE

This contributed chapter was accepted for publication in this refereed edited volume on June 26, 2021.

REFERENCE

"Indian hotel industry takes over Rs 1.30 lakh cr revenue hit in FY21, seeks govt support: FHRAI," *The Economic Times*, 16 May 2021, https://economictimes.indiatimes.com/industry/services/hotels-/-restaurants/indian-hotel-industry-takes-over-rs-1-30-lakh-cr-revenue-hit-in-fy21-seeks-govt-support-fhrai/articleshow/82676918.cms?from=mdr.

VIRTUAL FIRESIDE CONVERSATIONS WITH PROFESSIONALS AND BUSINESS LEADERS

With Co-editors Aurobindo Ghosh (AG), Amit Haldar (AH), and Kalyan Bhaumik (KB)

Conversation with **Subhobroto Chakroborty (SC), Founder and CEO, The Digital Guy, discussed the impact of COVID-19 on education, jobs, e-commerce, and finally, digital marketing**.

1 **The pandemic has affected almost all businesses, some like leisure, hospitality, and travel, worse than others. How has digital marketing been affected, in terms of growth or decline, by the pandemic?**

SC: Digital marketing has been growing since the pandemic. There are more people than ever believing in its power. At a personal level, I have seen more businesses approach me to work on their brands and businesses, particularly the ones who had put digital marketing on hold. Additionally, I have had people approach me to work with them on their personal branding. Businesses and individuals alike are thinking about investing in digital marketing because they have seen the potential of having digital assets, as COVID-19 shut down many traditional businesses within six months, last year.

DOI: 10.4324/9781003218807-22

2 Two common features of the mitigation measures adopted by policymakers are social distancing and movement restrictions. Both have deleterious impacts on traditional retail. How has e-commerce evolved?

SC: E-commerce has boomed. Millions of electronic devices, mobile phones, laptops, and tablets were sold because schools, tuitions, and offices began to operate remotely. And everyone had to buy these online. E-commerce benefitted the most because of this.

So, first electronic devices. Then other, better devices. Those who already had laptops now wanted bigger screens to work on.

Not only were all e-commerce platforms doing very well in terms of sales, a lot of them saw a sharp increase in purchase of memberships and other loyalty programmes that offered the benefits of earlier, speedy delivery.

3 With more corporate communications and customer service happening online, have most companies adopted a coherent digital strategy?

SC: The one big change that happened was that customer service employees were asked to work from home. But that's not surprising because there was no other option. Shifting to remote work hardly deserves to be called a coherent digital strategy.

India announced a lockdown unexpectedly. It did not happen in a phased manner. So, most businesses did not get much time to shift to the digital setup properly.

Those who had invested in the digital infrastructure before the pandemic were prepared to handle all kinds of emergencies and were also able to adapt to the new demands and the new ecosystem mindfully. The others are still struggling. So, no, most companies haven't been able to adopt a coherent digital strategy.

4 One thing about headship is a pipeline in management positions and growing digital marketing, possibly social media and analytics as a career choice. Are young graduates ready for the changing world? What needs to happen to prepare them?

SC: Yes, positions at senior levels in digital marketing, social media marketing, and analytics are opening up. These are becoming feasible career choices.

While a computer would be preferable for online classes, a smartphone could also serve the purpose. However, the phone might be convenient for apps, but not for carrying out lengthy assignments or research. While 24% Indians own a smartphone, only 11% of households possess any type of computer, which includes desktop computers, laptops, notebooks, netbooks, palmtops, or tablets.

Even the penetration of digital technologies in India has been haphazard and exclusionary. According to the 2017–2018 National Sample Survey report on education, only 24% of Indian households have an internet facility. While 66% of India's population live in villages, only a little over 15% of rural households have access to internet services. In urban households, the proportion is 42% (Kundu, 2020).

In fact, only 8% of all households with members aged between five and 24 have both a computer and an internet connection. The digital divide is evident across class, gender, region, or place of residence. Among the poorest 20% households, only 2.7% have access to a computer and 8.9% to internet facilities. In the case of the top 20% households, the proportions are 27.6% and 50.5% (Kundu, 2020).

Education is in crisis at the moment. Schools and college campuses have been closed through 2020 due to an increasing number of COVID cases. This could even extend to 2021. Can we ensure the safety and security of our students, teachers, and staff? How do we discipline students? How can we protect older teachers? Will testing be available at every school and college? How do we redesign classrooms? Do we have supplies for the schools? Can we afford to pay teachers without students? Can parents afford to pay fees without work? There are many unanswered questions.

5 How can digital marketing enable companies to give back by defining the purpose of companies adopting such strategies?

SC: Purpose is as important as ever. Digital marketing companies, I bet, won't be able to do much here. They are equivalent to advertising agencies. And ad agencies receive briefs from clients. Brands hire them to do their digital marketing. Just as ad agencies don't help except the top brands, digital marketing agencies too won't help companies, especially in terms of defining their purpose.

Only 1% of the companies in India can afford ad agencies, digital agencies, performance agencies, marketing automation agencies, SEO agencies, UX/UI agencies, Web or app management agencies, mobile marketing agencies, email marketing agencies, media buying, and BTL.

In fact, that's the reason why when I founded my company. I did not make it a digital marketing company. We are consultants. Knowledge drive is not creative.

Digital marketing can help but digital marketing companies cannot, and should not, help companies by defining their purpose. On the contrary, digital marketing should have its strategy based on the business's purpose.

NOTE

This contributed chapter was accepted for publication in this refereed edited volume on June 28, 2021.

REFERENCE

Kundu, P., (2020), "Indian education can't go online – only 8% of homes with young members have computer with net link," https://scroll.in/article/960939/indian-education-cant-go-online-only-8-of-homes-with-school-children-have-computer-with-net-link.

EPILOGUE

The Unknown Unknowns and Residual Impact in a Post-COVID-19 World

Aurobindo Ghosh, Amit Haldar, and Kalyan Bhaumik

INTRODUCTION

This volume has probably raised more questions than answers from a multi-faceted perspective. Going forward, we want to capture the sentiments of the expert contributors of the *Unknown unknowns* about the future of this disease (Clark, 2017). Whether like smallpox or polio we would be able to eradicate or eliminate it completely, like measles we will have a regular vaccination protocol, or like the seasonal flu, COVID-19 would become an endemic and we have to live with it with appropriate testing, therapy, and vaccination envisioned in Singapore and the United Kingdom (Gan et al., 2021; John and Gan, 2021). These possible unknown future scenarios of health and well-being, only time will tell. For us, we would like to look at the denouement of the volume as probably a beginning of future explorations of this unique pandemic that brought the entire planet to its knees. Let us hear it in the contributors' own words.

STRATEGIC AND ECONOMIC PERSPECTIVES

On Post-Pandemic Universities and Future of Management Education

… While the pandemic itself will probably only leave a scar in the long run, the questions that it has asked of universities are existential. In particular, how will the modern, 'internationalised' university evolve in response to geopolitical changes and rising parochialism?

(Kong and Patra, Chapter 2)

Covid-19 has unwrapped the potential asset value of Management Education to society due to the widespread acceptance and stronger appreciation of blended/hybrid learning in education, across the board. Quality universities …managed to democratize management education and make it more inclusive, using a creative mix of hybrid and in-person delivery at a better tuition price point.

(Ghosh and Thomas, Chapter 3)

ON THE ECONOMIC AND POLICY IMPACT

Martin Luther King wrote, 'We are caught in an inescapable network of mutuality, …Whatever affects one directly, affects all indirectly.' Will the pandemic make us appreciate that we are all in it together, and that deep global cooperation and coordination is needed to deal with generational challenges like pandemic and climate change…

(Baig, Chapter 4)

MEDICAL PERSPECTIVE AND CHALLENGES

On Emergency Response and Human Conditions

The NYC experience brought into spotlight the weaknesses that are currently inherent in the US health care system … it would be an oversight not to recognize and continue to strengthen these vulnerabilities.

(Mukherjee, Deshwal and Bhatt, Chapter 9)

ON TESTING PROTOCOLS AND MANDATES

Serological tests—that detect antibodies—against the virus become positive only after the infection subsides. So, while "Universal Testing" and "Immunity/Vaccine passports" seem to be attractive propositions to detect all cases and isolate them, this may be practically impossible due to resource and financial constraints.

(Haldar, Chapter 7)

… updated scientific evidence will help to understand the complexities associated with COVID-19 herd immunity and the pathway to achieve it, if at all plausible.

(Ghosh, Goyal and Singh, Chapter 10)

Our results suggest that a combination of high rate of testing and rapid vaccination is very effective in bringing the pandemic under control quickly and economically.

(Bhattacharjee, Liao, Paul and Chaudhuri, Chapter 5)

Until herd immunity from COVID-19 is achieved through a combination of vaccination and recovery from infection, the usage of mask is highly recommended.

(Nandy, Chapter 8)

ON TESTING STRATEGIES, THERAPEUTICS, AND LABS

… my greatest learning has been to find preventive measures and be very diligent in following practices that prevent infection… I strongly believe conservative approach in most patients is appropriate.

(Roy Chowdhury, Chapter 11.1)

There must be an elaborate plan to vaccinate 40–60 crore (400–600 million) people [in India]. That would need 1.2 billion doses of vaccine. The rich should pay for the poor.

(Chatterjee, Chapter 11.2)

HUMAN ELEMENTS AND BUSINESS CONDITIONS

On Human Conditions and Jurisprudence

Against this background of a worldwide public health crisis, countless individual households afflicted with marital discord are undergoing their own unique personal crises…more adaptive couples have been able to reduce interpersonal conflict… simply by practising enhanced self-awareness…

(Bhaumik, Chapter 12)

…[The Pandemic] has thrown up myriad challenges to mankind. Judiciary had to adapt itself and in areas make paradigm course corrections to meet the aspirations of the society and fulfil the Constitutional mandates.

(Basak, Chapter 14)

ON THE FUTURE OF BUSINESS AND SMALL AND MEDIUM ENTERPRISES (SMES)

Industries are unwilling to adopt any new business model that needs major investment and at the moment, we can just wait and watch without definite conclusions.

(Srivastav, Chapter 15)

As a responsible member of the civil society, the author realised that paying it forward, particularly in giving to the underprivileged of society might be the best way to normalise humanity in what is now widely known as the new normal.

(Bhattacharya, Chapter 16)

In the short run, hotel owners have to make money through pandemic created opportunities. But overall, I think the hospitality industry will bounce back quite strongly…

(Bose, Chapter 17.1)

The idea of investing in more content and more digital assets is here to stay…A leader has got to know how to define…[Strategies] that can be recalibrated frequently to adapt to the changes that keep happening.

(Chakroborty, Chapter 17.2)

ON SPORTS AND RECREATION INDUSTRY

[In May 2021, India is] in the middle of the second wave and that also is going down in terms of numbers all around the country and most importantly, around the world. We need to get back to normalcy, that's what we live for and that's all what we want.

(Ganguly, Chapter 5)

THE CLOUDS OF CONCERN

Dark clouds of proliferation of falsehoods, intolerance, over-stretched health infrastructure, medical particularly vaccine inequity, pandemic restrictions fatigue, protectionism have been hovering over this lonely planet.

(Aurobindo Ghosh, Chapter 1)

Mankind's destiny is to stand or fall together.

(Datta-Ray, Chapter 13)

DENOUEMENT AND THE LIGHT AHEAD

As we planned to complete the book towards the end of December 2021, little did we know what was in store for us. The failure of COVAX and vaccine inequality between the different parts of the world led the world to another catastrophe. G20 countries received 15 times more COVID-19 vaccine doses per capita than countries in Sub-Saharan Africa. (Unicef Press release 27.10.21).

A novel variant of SARS-COV2, the Omicron (B.1.1.529) was first reported from South Africa in November 2021. It spread rapidly through the globe. The Omicron variant had a total of 60 mutations compared to the reference/ancestral variant. What was of concern was that 32 of these involved the Spike protein, the main antigenic target of antibodies generated by infections and many of the vaccines. This allowed the variant to escape the immunity generated by vaccination and natural infections. It was soon found to be more infectious, but less virulent. The deeper lung tissues were relatively spared, and case fatality rate was lower compared to the previous variants. This gave rise to the hope that natural infection with the Omicron virus will lead to the elusive "herd immunity" across the globe. On the flip side, higher infectiousness led to more rapid spread and tended to overwhelm the existing health structure. Self testing with Antigen Rapid Tests (e.g. lateral flow immunoassay) is becoming increasingly popular worldwide.

Two more sublineages of the Omicron BA1 variant, the BA2 and BA3 have also been described. Certain mutations in Omicron variant led to reduced sensitivity in a N-gene or S-gene genetic target for detection. S-gene target failure (SGTF)-causing deletion (Δ69-70) can be utilized by q PCR tests to rapidly detect a case as an Omicron (or Alpha) variant. The BA2 variant (or so-called "stealth variant") on the other hand lacks this SGTF and needs full sequencing for identification.

One interesting hypothesis behind the emergence of this Omicron variant from Africa has been the coexistence of untreated HIV patients with poor immunity allowing the SARS-COV2 to mutate. No wonder the WHO warns of newer variants emerging in the days to come unless we put our heads together.

Amit Haldar (February 2022)

The decline in infections from the Delta variant and the nascent global economic recovery suddenly staggered to a saunter with the Omicron variant that South African Scientists did a phenomenal job identifying and alerting the world in November of 2021. Question was whether it was the beginning of the end or the end of the beginning of the pandemic? While the apparent lack of virulence of the Omicron strain was good news for the vaccinated, but higher transmissibility still disrupted global trade, commerce and movement besides having health costs for the unvaccinated and vulnerable. Indeed, continued push towards vaccination helped contain the virulence of the disease, and rollout of boosters helped keep immunity up. Although the global economy is not out of the woods yet. Economic toll of the pandemic includes the increasing inequity in access to resources and medicine, which might have been one of the main causes on the rise of the omicron strain. Higher inflation risk which also inordinately impacts the less privileged part of the society might have been a consequence of continued supply chain disruptions like chip shortage and higher freight costs. Finally, civil strife like farmer protests in India and the truckers strike in Canada also reflects the widening fissures in the society. '…All for one and one for all, united we stand divided we fall…' is not just the battle cry of the Three Musketeers in Alexandre Dumas' eponymous classical novel, it might be the solution for countries and the world to get back on a sustained path of growth.

Aurobindo Ghosh (February 2022)

REFERENCES

Clark, D., (2017), "Simple ways to spot unknown unknowns," *Harvard Business Review*, June 23, 2017, https://hbr.org/2017/10/simple-ways-to-spot-unknown-unknowns.

Gan, K. Y., L. Wong and Y. K. Ong, (2021), "Living normally, with Covid-19: Task force ministers on how S'pore is drawing road map for new normal," *The Straits Times*, June 24, 2021, https://www.straitstimes.com/opinion/living-normally-with-covid-19.

John, T. and N. Gan, (2021), "Singapore and the UK are both planning to 'live with Covid.' They are worlds apart on how to do that," 17 July, 2021, https://edition.cnn.com/2021/07/16/asia/singapore-uk-covid-reopening-intl-hk-gbr/index.html.

INDEX

Note: **Bold** page numbers refer to tables; *italic* page numbers refer to figures.

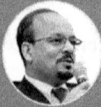
Aurobindo Ghosh
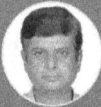
Amit Haldar
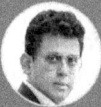
Kalyan Bhaumik
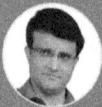
Sourav Ganguly
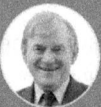
Howard Thomas
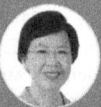
Lily Kong

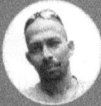
Sovan Patra
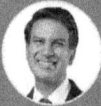
Taimur Baig
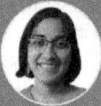
Satarupa Bhattacharjee
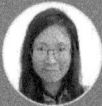
Shuting Liao
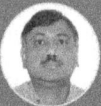
Debashis Paul
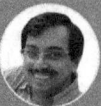
Sanjay Chaudhuri

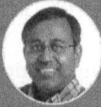
Rajesh Nandy
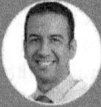
Vikramjit Mukherjee
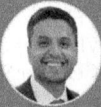
Himanshu Deshwal
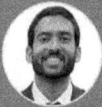
Alok Bhatt
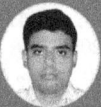
Arnab Ghosh
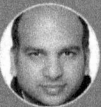
Kapil Goyal

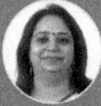
Mini P Singh
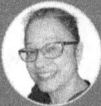
S RoyChowdhury
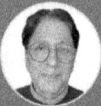
, Somenath Chatterjee
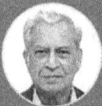
Sunanda K Datta-Ray
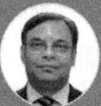
Debangsu Basak
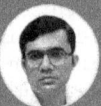
Anurag Srivastava

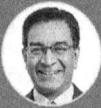
Ajay bhattacharya
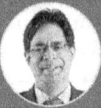
Suborno Bose
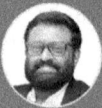
Subhobroto Chakraborty
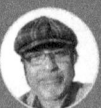
Partha Bhattacharjee

For Product Safety Concerns and Information please contact our EU
representative GPSR@taylorandfrancis.com
Taylor & Francis Verlag GmbH, Kaufingerstraße 24, 80331 München, Germany